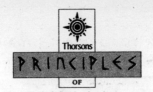

Thorsons
PRINCIPLES
OF

AYURVEDA

ANNE GREEN

Thorsons

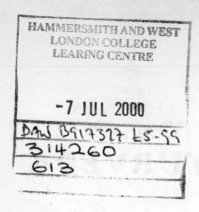
Thorsons
An Imprint of HarperCollins*Publishers*
77–85 Fulham Palace Road
Hammersmith, London W6 8JB

The Thorsons website address is: www.thorsons.com

Published by Thorsons 2000
1 3 5 7 9 10 8 6 4 2

© Anne Green 2000

Anne Green asserts the moral right to
be identified as the author of this work

A catalogue record for this book
is available from the British Library

ISBN 0 7225 3745 X

Printed and bound in Great Britain by
Caledonian International Book Manufacturing Ltd, Glasgow

314260

CONTENTS

ACKNOWLEDGEMENTS

T hanks in deepest gratitude to my teachers Dr Vasant Lad and Dr Robert Svoboda for planting seeds and encouraging growth. They taught me that Ayurveda embodies laws of nature that are unvarying, eternal and non-culturally specific. I therefore accept all responsibility for any distortions of the true teachings in my interpretations.

Special thanks to my friend and yoga teacher Clair Stevens for her help with the section on yoga postures. Finally, my love and appreciation to Jude Glendinning, Judith Morrison, Angela Hope-Murray, Deborah Tickner, Rowena Ardern, Jayne Woollam, David Green and my family for their varied, invaluable and sustaining support.

PUBLISHERS' NOTE

This is a reference work. It is not meant for diagnosis or treatment and it is not a substitute for consultation with a duly-licensed health care professional.

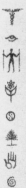

FOREWORD

I t is harder than ever today for us to know exactly who we are. If the Internet is bringing the world into the sharpest focus yet for some, others have gone missing in the information-jungle. Ask one question and you can be swamped with often-conflicting answers; lose your bearings in cyber-space and until you find them again you will wander aimless in a mapless Web.

Learning to 'locate' ourselves is clearly the need of the hour. We will be able to keep our heads when all about us are losing theirs only when we have clear ideas what those heads can and cannot do for us. Some people have a natural aptitude for mathematics, a 'head for numbers', but have two left feet; others cannot multiply or divide to save their lives but seem to have been born to dance. When we know our heads we can know which way we are heading, we can orient ourselves even when our environment is disoriented.

Ayurveda, India's ancient system of wholistic living, was developed long ago to help people understand who they are, what they should be doing in life, and how they should be doing it. Ayurveda focuses on self-discovery, self-knowledge, and self-definition. It organizes its knowledge into theories of health and disease that speak eloquently to all listeners of life's basic rules, how those rules can be used to maintain and enhance health, and how to use them to retrieve health that has been compromised by disease. Ayurveda teaches people how to learn about themselves, that they may live life with a maximum of enjoyment and a minimum of misery.

The cacophony in the medical marketplace, where techniques, therapies and supplements clamour loudly for our attention, can confuse even the experts. Ayurveda values introspection over appetite; it advises to look first inside to discover what your organism truly requires rather than to decide what to eat or wear or read or do on the basis of hungers and thirsts alone. All foods and remedies are good for some people some of the time, but nothing is appropriate for everyone at all times. Learn more of who you are and you will know more of what is appropriate for you; live appropriately and you will find yourself living as healthily as you possibly can.

Ayurveda depends on no particular culture or era for its understanding of embodied life; anyone from anywhere can benefit from its wisdom, so long as that wisdom is judiciously and accurately communicated. Anne Green, the author of this volume, has studied Ayurveda extensively for many years, and both Dr Vasant Lad and I greatly appreciate her contribution to this enormous work of making its wisdom available to a modern audience. Consider her words thoughtfully, apply them in the context of your own life, and it will not be long before you will see what this ancient art of living can do for you.

Dr Robert G. Svoboda

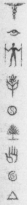

INTRODUCTION: WHAT IS AYURVEDA?

THE SCIENCE OF DAILY LIFE

Ayurveda is the ancient Indian healing system and life science.

The word Ayurveda is a Sanskrit term meaning science of daily life or longevity, from two roots: *ayus* meaning 'life', 'daily living' or 'life cycle', and *vid* meaning 'knowledge', 'path' or 'science'.

Ayurveda is both a science and an art as it contains wisdom about how to thrive as a psychological, emotional and spiritual being as well as knowledge about body functions and disease processes. Intuition is regarded as an innate human faculty that can be used with awareness, and by constant use, developed into a peerless and sensitive sounding device for diagnosis, prognosis and prescribing.

Ayurveda's deep roots began long before there was a script to record them; mnemonic verses – chanted phrases comprising lists of herbs with particular actions, or signs and symptoms of particular types of imbalance – were the means by which traditions were passed down from master to pupil. This enabled masses of information to be absorbed and retained.

Ayurveda is an 'energetic' system, which means that it categorizes according to the energies that characterize things and the qualities they exhibit. For example, it is meaningful within Ayurveda that a certain food exerts a predominantly heating rather than a cooling effect upon a person who eats it – that food is said to have heating energy. This also applies to individuals: a person with a very creative imagination who is easily spooked, has a slim body, poor digestion and skin that tans easily will be categorized differently from someone who is rather phlegmatic and ultra calm, heavily built, with slow and extremely efficient digestion and pale, cool skin. This is in obvious contrast to systems of medicine where substances that comprise the *Materia Medica* are analysed in terms of chemical constituents, and where the qualities used to describe people are restricted to their symptoms, without taking into consideration their body type or characteristics.

WHOLISM OF TRADITIONAL INDIAN KNOWLEDGE

As one of the main traditional systems of the Indian subcontinent (and Sri Lanka), Ayurveda has been in existence for thousands of years. The knowledge it imparts has evolved (with some relatively abrupt additions and subtractions) through historical, cultural and religious change. The changes it has undergone reflect the strength of a flexible system and have always been congruent with the spirit and philosophy of the myth of its Divinely inspired inception.

The story of ancient seers being gathered together in the Himalayas to decide how humanity's ills could best be addressed, of their receiving the laws of nature as Divine revelation from the god Indra, underlies the precept that Ayurveda is eternal. The truth about human life made manifest in the science of life is always the same – seers, those who 'see' (the truth), will always be able to deduce these laws. Therefore, even without any living tradition Ayurveda would be accessible to such beings, in any culture, at any time.

Ayurveda is one of the three great Vedic life sciences, the other two being Yoga and Tantra. Each of these has a different main perspective on human life, while accepting the importance of the others. All three address what is necessary and sufficient to live a healthy life. The word 'healthy' means 'hale' or 'whole'. To be whole we need to have balance within and between body, mind and spirit, since all of these are part of what it means to be human.

WHAT'S YOUR TYPE?

The main focus of Ayurveda is on the physical aspect of existence; the body is the vehicle for our Divine spark which travels within through the world of Mammon. Without the body we cannot experience through the senses, and without good health it is much more difficult to enjoy our span on earth and to give our attention to concerns of the spirit and finding our way 'home', back to the Oneness from whence we, and everything, came.

How can we be healthy if we do not know what to aim for? Health is more than freedom from disease, and is something to do with balance and strength. But, since each of us is unique, how do we proceed?

Phrases like 'the constitution of an ox' point us towards the crucial concept. We all know, if not first-hand then by reputation, the ideal of a strong constitution which confers on those blessed with the ability to withstand the ravages of early 21st-century environmental, social and personal pressures. In Ayurveda, a balanced individual constitution is the key to health. Having an awareness of what you are fundamentally gives shape to your endeavours to improve. In this text you

will find ways to assess both your constitution and what is
awry, and some help with what to do about it.

WHAT SORT OF STUFF ARE WE MADE OF?

Behind the idea of constitution (something one is born with)
are more profound questions like what are we made of, how
have we come to be as we are, and why are we made this way?
Ayurveda, being the science of life, addresses these questions.

THE FIVE ELEMENTS

The physical universe and everything in it is comprised of the
five great elements:

Ether   can express itself as the space within which everything
        exists and the space(s) within everything
Air   can express itself as the gaseous state of matter
Fire   can express itself as transformational energy
Water   can express itself as the liquid state of matter
Earth   can express itself as the solid state of matter

Within the body structure formed by these elements, function
is governed by three energies or humours, known in the
Ayurvedic tradition as *Doshas*:

• Vata
• Pitta
• Kapha

There is more about these three Doshas in Chapter 3 and
throughout this book, but for now they can be briefly summa-
rized as follows:

The Vata energy is a composite of the elements of Air and Ether, and is characterized by being erratic, cold, active, dry, clear and subtle.

The Pitta energy is a composite of the elements of Fire and Water, is characterized by being intense, hot, oily and sharp.

The Kapha energy is a composite of the elements of Water and Earth, is characterized by being calm, heavy, cool and moist.

The balance or imbalance of these three Doshas in our lives determines health or dis-ease. Our individual constitutions (physical, mental and emotional) reflect a personal and unique mix of Vata, Pitta and Kapha.

GETTING THE BLEND RIGHT

The unique blend of Vata, Pitta and Kapha that is you comes into being as a result of the mixture in your parents at the time of conception. If your parents were trying to find a new home and your mother worked as an international air stewardess prior to your conception and insisted on decorating the whole house in time for your arrival, she might well have contributed mostly Vata to your constitution. Father's career as a professional musician might have been in the doldrums about this time, leaving him rather low in spirits and anxious about the future, so that his contribution towards your constitution might also have been rather Vata-ish. That you are now likely to score high on Vata in the Constitution Questionnaire (see pages 57–61) is understandable. Your individual blend of Vata, Pitta and Kapha is the sum of what is predominant in both parents at the time of conception. Mother's activities, diet, emotions during pregnancy and any perinatal events such as a Caesarean or induced birth will also affect your constitution.

Throughout life, your own choices and experiences, from diet and exercise to your taste in music and films will in turn affect and be affected by the balance of these energies within you. Ayurveda points out that everything: food, medicine, time of day, stage of life, season of the year, colour ... must, by virtue of its being made of the same 'stuff' (elements) as we are, affect the balance of Vata, Pitta and Kapha within us. Use with awareness what you eat, think, look at and indulge in to balance the three energies and thus participate in co-creating your own fate.

HEALTH AND DISEASE

How health is defined by a society and how it experiences disease is dependent upon what the main culture considers what it means to be human. In our materialistic West, the dominant culture sees body and mind as, for the most part, separate and independent, because that was the pronouncement of early scientific investigators; human bodies are seen as intricate and complex mechanisms that need fixing when they malfunction.

Cultures that see human beings as an integral part of the great universe view disease and health as, respectively, imbalance and the restoration of a dynamic balance – within a person's body, mind and spirit, and between that person and his or her environment. You will find that Ayurveda's theories of health and disease resonate deep within, because we humans have an innate sense of being part of the greater whole.

Disease is seen as the outcome of imbalance of the Vata, Pitta or Kapha energies. Any of these can become excessive by the principle of 'like increases like' (its corollary being 'unlike decreases excess'). If you are already experiencing an increase in Vata (like the high-flying mother described above), then you

need to adjust your lifestyle (diet, exercise and socializing) to
calm the spiralling Vata.

A BALANCED LIFE

Ayurveda has much to offer you. Think of a balanced life as a
beautiful patchwork quilt. Many pieces can be put in various
places to produce an effective design – so is it with some of the
therapies and activities you will read about in this book. The
centrepiece of your quilt, however, is not something that can be
placed anywhere other than the centre, and so it is with design-
ing a healthy life: diet, lifestyle and the more subtle emotional
and spiritual needs are of central importance. Stitch well!

AYURVEDA'S HISTORY AND ORIGINS

Most humans have an understandable fascination with our origins as a species and culture. Related to this is the equally understandable but unfortunate belief that everything with a long history is unquestionably valuable and undeniably right. It is as if our powers of discrimination switch off when we hear the words 'ancient lineage' or even 'prehistoric antecedents'.

Now, I can endorse the line of argument that says that if a system of thought has survived for millennia then it is likely to contain significant truths. However, before we start in on the history of Ayurveda I want to record my belief that the proof of the Ayurvedic pudding is definitely in the eating. Many people writing about Ayurveda have pandered to this 'ancient antecedents' fallacy and it is just not necessary. Ayurveda works as it has evolved and developed and not just because of the age of its origins.

EARLY INDUS VALLEY CIVILIZATION

From approximately 3500 BC in the valley of the Indus River, in what is present-day Pakistan, factors like the fertility of the land and the growth of trade gave birth to a civilization responsible for the city-states Harappa, Mohenjo-daro and the port of Lothal. At the height of its flowering, from about 3000 to 1500 BC, these had all the accoutrements of a highly developed culture including well-constructed roads, plumbing and drainage systems.

THE ARYANS AND THE VEDAS

Climatic and environmental changes, and also devastation due to increasing invasion by the Aryans (nomadic peoples from Central Asia) caused the eventual demise of the Indus culture. The Aryans brought with them the *Vedas* (from Sanskrit, meaning 'the knowledge') – rituals, hymns, prayers to and praise of the gods responsible for health, fertility and longevity, transmitted as an oral tradition.

Disease and healing were mostly dealt with indirectly in the Vedas – gods were ascribed healing powers, diseases were often seen as the works of malefic spirits, while injuries and broken bones were regarded as having more commonplace causes. As in Egyptian medicine, magic, faith-healing and herbs were all valued therapeutic tools.

There are four Vedas. Atharva-Veda is the youngest of the four and is made up of more than 100 hymns on the subject of health, disease and healing. The other Vedic texts contain in comparison but few of such references.

Ayurveda is regarded as a subsidiary of the Atharva-Veda. This said, it is important to state that there was no system of Vedic medicine *per se*, and that if Ayurveda has antecedents in the Atharva-Veda text then it also owes something to other traditions.

AYURVEDA AND EARLY BUDDHISM

The new religious groups of the second half of the 1st millennium
BC (with particular reference to that of Gautama Sakyamuni,
the Buddha) also contributed to the development of Ayurveda by
the common process of cross-fertilization. The famous physician
Jivaka, who was appointed by King Bimbisara to tend to the
Buddha and his community, is reputed to have given Buddha an
Ayurvedic purgative at his request. So many ill people asked to
join the community with the express purpose of being treated by
Jivaka that eventually it was decided that those already ill would
have to be excluded from seeking membership.

The Buddhist canonical texts and later Ayurvedic texts
indicate that there developed parallels in treatment and medicinal substances. The Buddhist communities developed rather
sophisticated facilities, which by about 250 BC extended
beyond treating the monks to include the laity.

THE SOURCE TEXTS

During the 1st millennium BC the main texts still used in
Ayurveda today appeared: the Charaka Samhita (The Wander-
er's Compendium) and Sushruta Samhita (Charaka and
Sushruta being the names of the respective authors of these
works; Samhita meaning 'compendium'). Both have been
reworked over time by other writers with other interpretations
or axes to grind; additions and changes have been made.
Charaka's text has more passages of theory and philosophical
discourse, while Sushruta's has detailed descriptions of surgical techniques, some of which do not appear in Charaka's at all.

Although precise dating is only possible from the lifetime
of the Buddha (563–483 BC), early versions of the Charaka
Samhita (the older of the two) probably date from about that

time. The version in contemporary use has alterations by writers of the second half of the 1st millennium AD. Alterations to Shushruta's text continued until much later.

Both of these texts are weighty tomes. The 120 chapters of the Charaka Samhita alone contain about three times the volume of surviving Hippocratic medical texts; and translations of Shushruta are even longer.

Other writers, such as Vagbhata (approximately 600 AD) wrote almost 2,000 years after Charaka and Sushruta. Vagbhata's text (Ashtanga Hrydaya) is considered to have extracted the essence of the earlier teachings, which accounts for its popularity among those studying Ayurveda as a life system today.

TRADITION AND CONTINUITY

Both Charaka and Sushruta constructed their concepts from the same philosophical foundations, mainly using constructs found in what is now known as Samkhya philosophy (discussed in detail in Chapter 2). It is interesting to note that Charaka's contribution actually predates the core texts of the Samkhya school of philosophy.

It is also a source of debate that, although Sushruta wrote in great detail about surgical training and procedures, there is little evidence of such skilled operations being carried out in subsequent generations; that is until the famous 'nose job' of March 1793. Two British surgeons watched this plastic surgery being performed and a detailed account was published in London the following year, along with diagrams. This led to the adoption of the 'Hindu method' in Western plastic surgery as it was far superior to anything known at that time in the West.

The Indian medical tradition (in common with all indigenous systems of medicine) has always had common streams and a classical tradition. Folk medicine took (and still takes) different forms in various parts of the country. Herbal treatment for common diseases is often practised by women and passed on from mother to daughter. Various other skills like bone-setting, ear-wax picking and massage have been the field of expertise of particular groups or individuals who have kept specific skills alive through the years and introduced new techniques and knowledge.

Also, Ayurvedic texts, unlike modern medical texts, are written versions of what was, for an inordinately long time, passed down orally and retained only in the memory. The Ayurvedic material contained the distilled essence of the subject under discussion. Chapters ended with summarizing verses that could be more easily remembered than prose and which could trigger the student's or practitioner's memory of related material. This, given the innate creativity of our thought processes (when not restricted by concepts of an absolutely right or wrong answer), led and still leads to new, useful and insightful ideas. That each practitioner would and should treat in an individualized way is therefore endorsed by the Ayurvedic perspective.

Thus, for these several and varied reasons it may have been that by observation and demonstration the skill of rhinoplasty was passed down within particular groups (the 'surgeon' who performed the recorded surgery was of the brickmakers' caste) and that it changed and developed outside of the classical profession. Ayurveda was and is a dynamic tradition.

Another possible factor in the apparent disappearance of Ayurvedic surgery after Sushruta's evident knowledge and practise of it is the belief held by the Brahmans (the high caste of priests and men of learning) that any touching of the body or its emanations was a defilement for the Vaidya (Ayurvedic physician).

The caste system that emerged from the Aryan Vedic culture once settlement in the Indian subcontinent was established was based on one's degree of involvement in life's daily round. The lower castes were deemed so because they undertook tasks of the most physical kind, such as cleaning and digging. Those who belonged to the highest castes (priests and nobility) were not supposed to involve themselves in the aspects of life that reflected its gross (meaning both non-subtle and disgusting) nature.

AN AYURVEDIC PHYSICIAN'S TRAINING

Traditionally, a person who desired to become a physician would first consider the suitability of his own character and personality to undertake such a profession. He sought to balance the benefits of remuneration and fulfilment against the demands of the vocation. Having decided to pursue this career, the student would then decide upon which of the classical texts to study and seek out a guru as an essential part of the equation. The selection of a guru by the pupil was followed by the guru's imposing a probationary period of six months during which he decided whether or not he agreed basically with the student's self-assessment of suitability to the profession. The guru's role was to extrapolate on the text, to flesh out the bones of the teachings, exemplify by practice and to inspire his students.

A close personal bond was essential as the combination of respect and love was a powerful motivation to the student to pursue his studies vigorously. The student often lived as a member of the guru's family until deemed to have internalized Ayurveda to the satisfaction of the guru. Tuition was free, but upon completion the new physician would bring, at his guru's request, an appropriate gift.

Frequent meetings with other Vaidyas and their students to hone their intellectual skills and knowledge in debate introduced students to different interpretations of the text and helped prevent rigidity of outlook. The university at Takshashila (6th century BC) which produced the physician Jivaka would most likely have been a loosely connected group of gurus and their followers who met in the pursuit of their studies.

THE PEAK YEARS

From about 500 BC till the early centuries of the 1st millennium AD, Ayurveda was an integral science in a thriving culture. Apart from the Buddha's endorsement, there were other important personages who encouraged the Indian science of life.

Alexander the Great was sufficiently impressed with Ayurveda during his 4th-century BC invasion of northern India to give sole responsibility for treating poisoning to Vaidyas, and to take some of them with him on his departure.

In the 3rd century BC the Buddhist convert, Ashok, Emperor of northern India, set up hospitals and veterinary clinics throughout the region and sent abroad missionaries who also spread their medical knowledge.

The Buddhists set up campus universities at which the science and art of medicine was taught along with many other disciplines. Several more key Ayurvedic texts appeared during the same period, which ended with the Muslim invasions from the north and the subsequent attempted eradication of the Buddhists along with their culture, knowledge and institutions. The Buddhism fundamental to Ayurveda in Sri Lanka remains today. Also, the flight of Buddhist monks to Nepal and Tibet ahead of the invaders added to the already present influence of Ayurveda upon the traditional systems of medicine in these countries.

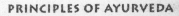

CULTURE AND POLITICS

The opening up and expansion of trade routes to India during the 16th and 17th centuries enabled Europeans to import its goods and knowledge. The romance with India continued while xenophobia increased, until there was a clamp-down on the transmission of Indian wisdom and knowledge.

In 1835, Lord Macaulay decreed that in all areas where the British East India Company held sway, only the teaching of Western knowledge would have official sanction. Thus the cross-cultural exchange of medical knowledge more or less ceased. Without the existence of official support, indigenous knowledge had few heirs and much was lost during the following years.

During the years leading up to Indian independence in 1947, Ayurveda received the support of nationalists due to the fact that it represented a uniquely Indian system of medicine. Since independence, the government has had the more difficult job of trying to marry its modern, Western-influenced views on bio-medicine with the pragmatics of governing a population for whom a huge part of daily life and cultural and spiritual life is saturated with Ayurvedic concepts and values.

Current governmental policy is to provide training in Ayurveda at specifically designated colleges and universities, and to include that system of medicine in its health policy. However, much less funding and far fewer facilities are provided for such training than is consonant with official governmental statements about the place of Ayurveda in the medical pantheon.

Many more Vaidyas practise in rural than urban areas, reflecting the type of communities that support Ayurveda. Also, few Vaidyas use solely traditional remedies. The infiltration of drugs and particularly injections (which seem to have a mystical and mythical fascination for many patients) into the traditional physician's repertoire is increasingly common. Patient demand, in part conditioned by contact with the West, is one reason for this. Another is the inclusion of some bio-medicine, public health and family planning in the curriculum of Ayurvedic colleges.

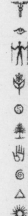

AYURVEDIC PHILOSOPHY AND COSMOLOGY

Ayurveda accepts that creation is the point at which any science of life must start, and therefore the philosophy of creation and cosmology is where we must begin. Philosophy is never the easiest part to understand of any system, and this goes for the philosophical foundations of Ayurveda. However, although it is essential to begin at the beginning it is not quite so essential to have a thorough grounding in Ayurvedic philosophy for the practical aspects of Ayurveda described later in this book to work for you. You might prefer to come back to this chapter as the desire grows in you to understand more of this comprehensive system of health care.

THE SIX PHILOSOPHIES

The philosophy of creation and cosmology chiefly endorsed by Ayurveda is Sankhya (from the Sanskrit roots *sat*, meaning 'truth', and *khya* which means 'to know'), established by the Vedic seer Kapila. Having said this, Ayurveda's philosophical foundations draw upon a range of six Vedic philosophies (or *Shad Darshan*):

- Sankhya
- Vedanta
- Vaisheshika
- Yoga
- Nyaya
- Mimansa

Each of these contributes to the total precepts of Ayurveda, and shares many concepts with the others.

Of these six philosophies, Sankhya is the best suited to conceptualizing the process of creation of the universe and all that is contained therein, including humankind. It outlines the process of creation from the subtlest energies to dense matter.

SANKHYA PHILOSOPHY OF CREATION

Sankhya philosophy speaks of the interrelationship of the cosmos and humanity ('as above, so below; as within, so without' – the idea that human beings mirror and are mirrored by the cosmos). Through meditation and revelation, the *rishis* (seers) perceived that the universe and all contained therein is the manifestation of the Divine/Pure Awareness.

Unlike the Judeo-Christian view of creation, which posits God as Creator of humankind (and the rest of the universe) in His image but not of His substance, the view taken by Ayurveda is of God and everything created by Him/Her as One. God, the non-material Source of everything, manifests as everything.

PURUSHA AND PRAKRUTI: THE TWO IN ONE

Purusha is the name given the original One, the Indivisible, Pure Awareness, the All-That-There-Is, the Singularity that spontaneously desires to experience Him/Herself.

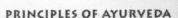

The desire to experience Him/Herself sows the seed of the universe which (with all its billions of components, organic and inorganic, sentient and more or less non-sentient) gradually emerges out of the void which contains all potentialities.

Though a unity, we have to think of Purusha as a polarity in order to understand how the universe is created – male and female, Shiva and Shakti, Purusha and Prakruti. Purusha is formless, attribute-less, choice-less, passive and is the non-participating witness to the Mother of Creation, Nature, Prakruti, as she chooses to manifest in billions of ways. Prakruti has attributes including form, colour and the will to make choices.

MAHAT: COSMIC INTELLIGENCE

From the initial polarity of witness and actor comes the first manifestation: Mahat, Cosmic Intelligence. Mahat is the reason there is order in the cosmos, 'everything in its place' from stars in galaxies to liver cells being produced in the right organ.

INDIVIDUAL INTELLIGENCE: AHAMKARA

Individual intelligence is seen as a stepping-down, a fragmentation of Prakruti as it manifests through Mahat to the individual level. This forms our own Higher Selves, our inner wisdom.

So, from Cosmic Intelligence comes individual intelligence, Ahamkara. Ahamkara is not the same as the 'ego' of Freudian psychoanalysis, but comes from Sanskrit terms that mean 'the I-maker'. Ahamkara contains everything that causes us to see ourselves as distinct individuals. It comprises all aspects of the self, including the knowledge of what parts of the universe are 'me' and what is 'other'. It is the organizing principle that enables every cell in the body to resonate with every other cell. All things in the universe have Ahamkara. Self-identification occurs and 'I' exists as separate from Mahat.

We are ultimately, inextricably one and the same. It is also true that to exist in this universe and remain functioning in our everyday existence, we must have ego. Even enlightened beings must have at least fragments of ego to remain alive as humans. All our ills as humans stem from our apparent separateness, our belief that we are discrete entities. Our spiritual quest is to rediscover our oneness.

Ahamkara, the 'I-maker', equates to some extent with the lower self. As soon as there is 'I', everything that is not 'I' becomes the 'other', the environment, the object to I's subject. Through this individualized expression of the Universal Consciousness, subjective and objective realities, organic and inorganic worlds and sentient and non-sentient beings manifest.

OBJECTIVE AND SUBJECTIVE REALITIES

There are three attributes, or *gunas*, which are inherent within Prakruti. These qualities are:

- Sattva (clarity, balance, truth)
- Rajas (movement, activity)
- Tamas (inertia, obstruction, resistance).

From a state of potentiality in Prakruti they emerge as qualities of Ahamkara, interacting to create the next 'stepping-down' or level down from Primordial Energy towards the material.

SATTVA

The subjectivity of Sattva ('I' as a sentient being with individual consciousness) gives rise to the five senses which take in information from the world (hearing, touch, sight, taste and smell) and also the five senses of action that enable us to make impressions upon the physical world (vocalizing, manual manipulation, locomotion, procreation and excretion). Sattva

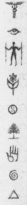

also creates mind which, of course, both receives sensory input and initiates action as well as being responsible for emotion and cognition.

RAJAS AND TAMAS

Rajas is the kinetic energy that enables Sattva to manifest its subjective world and Tamas to create the objective world of subtle and dense elements. The subtle elements are sound, touch, sight, taste and smell – the objects of Sattva's senses. The dense elements are Ether, Air, Fire, Water and Earth. Tamas is the primordial essence of matter; nothing material, from a nerve fibre to an oak tree, exists on the physical plane but by the presence of Tamas.

Using the word 'dense' in this context needs an explanation – it is the accepted term for the five elements, or *Mahabhutas*, but the common usage of 'dense' is certainly not what they represent. We are not talking of 'elements' in the sense of oxygen, hydrogen, nitrogen, etc. in the periodic table of elements, but of entities and forces that lie behind those things. So, 'dense' here is relative only to the finer, faster vibrations of other higher manifestations of the Mother of Creation.

The true nature of mind is Sattvic, but Rajas and Tamas are necessary so that the universe can exist as it does. There must be movement and there must be some stability. Without Rajas the whole of creation would not evolve; without Tamas it would be in a constant state of flux.

VARIATIONS ON A THEME

There are, as one would expect, different interpretations of and different schools of thought about Sankhya. It is often described as having 24 principles (or *Tattvas*), though some sources claim there are 25.

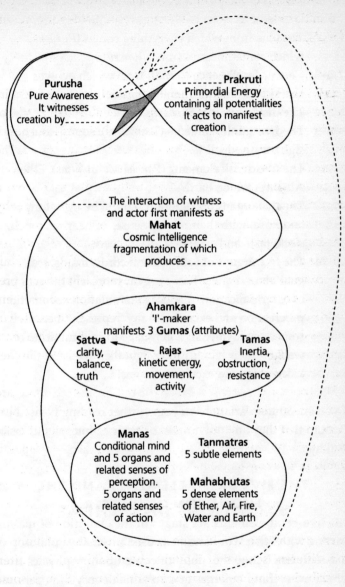

Purusha
Pure Awareness
It witnesses
creation by ....

Prakruti
Primordial Energy
containing all potentialities
It acts to manifest
creation ....

.... The interaction of witness
and actor first manifests as
Mahat
Cosmic Intelligence
fragmentation of which
produces ....

Ahamkara
'I'-maker
manifests 3 **Gumas** (attributes)
Sattva   ← **Rajas** →   **Tamas**
clarity,   kinetic energy,   Inertia,
balance,   movement,   obstruction,
truth   activity   resistance

Manas
Conditional mind
and 5 organs and
related senses of
perception.
5 organs and
related senses
of action

Tanmatras
5 subtle elements

Mahabhutas
5 dense elements
of Ether, Air, Fire,
Water and Earth

The 24 Principles of Sankhya Philosophy of Creation

PRINCIPLES OF AYURVEDA

Taking the 24-principle approach, they are as follows:

1   The One from which everything comes (*Purusha*, which sometimes subsumes *Prakruti*)

2–3   Cosmic Intelligence (*Mahat*) from which evolves individual identification (*Ahamkara*)

4   The discursive mind (*Manas*)

5–9   The five subtle elements (*Tanmatras*): sound, touch, sight, taste, smell

10–14   The five dense elements (*Pancha Mahabhutas*): Ether, Air, Fire, Water, Earth

15–19   The five organs of cognition: ears, skin, eyes, tongue and nose, with their related senses of hearing, touch, sight, taste and smell

20–24   The five organs of action: vocal cords, hands, feet, genitals and anus. These organs represent the actions of communication, manual manipulation, locomotion, procreation and excretion. I say 'represent' because someone may use sign language to communicate or walk on their hands rather than their feet, and the kidneys too are excretory organs!

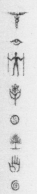

If you encounter variations in your further reading please bear in mind that they are individuals' or schools' interpretations of Sankhya.

THE FIVE GREAT ELEMENTS AND THE EVOLUTION OF MATTER

The five great elements are stages in the evolution of matter, starting with Ether. The concept as used in Sankhya philosophy is astoundingly like the 'field' of contemporary physics from which everything emerges and to which everything returns. Professor Ervin Laszlo, who was Science Advisor to the Director

> We are thinking of Ether as an informational medium. I am
> proposing a hypothesis which will look at the underlying energy
> field. The so-called vacuum is no longer a vacuum: it is fullness, a
> plenum. It is a virtual energy field which, however, has a very
> subtle effect on matter. It guides processes of development and
> evolution. In Hindu philosophy it is known as the Akashic
> Record.

Ether is the first manifestation on the physical plane of the cosmic, unsounded sound 'AUM' or 'OM'.

In this subtlest of mundane vibrations, the appearance of
movement is called **Air**. This Air produces friction, and friction
results in heat and accumulated heat produces **Fire** (which is
also light).

The outcome of Fire being applied to cosmic consciousness is
liquefaction of some of the principles therein, which is named
Water, and the consolidation and crystallization of some of
these principles is solid, is **Earth**, is matter.

THE ELEMENTS AS STATES OF MATTER

The five elements also represent states of matter:

- **Ether** represents space, the space that things take up and the
  space within them. Without space nothing can exist because
  it contains all potentialities and it bestows the freedom in
  which material and subtle entities (bodies and thoughts)
  exist and move.
- **Air** stands for all gaseous substances in the universe, not
  merely the (increasingly adulterated) mixture of gases that
  surrounds us and which we breathe.

- **Fire** is radiant heat and energy. Energy applied changes a substance, thus Fire is the transformative principle – it changes the state of substances, as when heat makes ice turn to water and water to steam.
- **Water** means everything in the universe that is in a liquid state.
- **Earth** represents all completely solid substances.

We can see that the five great elements are fundamental to the existence of the physical universe.

THE QUALITIES OF SENSORY EXPERIENCE

The qualitative nature of Ayurveda is complementary to the quantitative methods of Western science. 'Complementary' doesn't imply 'of secondary importance or value' in any sense. Several approaches may enhance one another; each fleshes out areas relatively neglected in the others. They can be seen as different views of a city from the mountaintops around it. From one peak alone the view is not fully comprehensive. A church tower blocks the view of the square behind it. From another vantage point, the square is seen and other features are obscured.

Ayurveda and its qualitative approach is a high mountain with a very extensive view. This is it functioning as a science. Add to that its power as an art, using the honed intuitive faculty, and you have an eagle arising from that peak with vision acute enough to fill in the information about the darkened corners of the city.

The Charaka Samhita lists 10 pairs of qualities traditionally seen as the foundation of our sensory experience. How something is affected by any of these qualities, how the quality shows up in things depends upon their interaction. For example, 'light' is one of the qualities on Charaka's list and it is defined as the power of yeast to make bread rise, the power of an air balloon to fly, and as the 'spaceyness' of someone who spends too much time at her computer!

THE 10 PAIRED QUALITIES

Light	Heavy
Moist/Oily	Dry
Rough	Smooth
Cold	Hot
Subtle	Gross
Clear	Cloudy
Soft	Hard
Stable/Static	Mobile
Solid	Liquid
Dull	Intense

These qualities describe the perceptual experience that we have of the physical world, so only the ranges of these qualities that affect human experience are of interest to us in a healing system. (For example, we can never experience absolute zero as a temperature.)

You will encounter these qualities again and again in your studies of Ayurveda, although sometimes synonyms are used for some of the terms given above. By reading and thinking about what you have read, these 10 polarities and the continuums they represent will start to describe meaningfully what you experience. You will start to associate them with yourself and everything and everyone you encounter. When that occurs, then you are in a position to affect your world, to change things. How and why will become apparent as we start to relate these qualities to our human bodies and our minds.

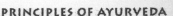

SUBTLE PHYSIOLOGY

From macrocosm to microcosm; 'as above, so below. As within, so without.' This aphorism encapsulates the Ayurvedic principle that everything in the external universe has its counterpart in the internal universe of the human body, mind and spirit.

This 'everything' includes, of course, the five great elements. The biological versions of these principles will not be identical to the elemental Ether, Air, Fire, Water and Earth, however. Just as a menu is not the meal and a map is not the actual territory, the blueprint for matter is not what actually exists in the physical.

- The human organism exists in space, which is another name for **Ether**. It also has numerous spaces within it and numberless spaces within the tiny organelles in all its cells.
- **Air** manifests as all movements of the body and within it – the microscopic pulsation of cells and the contractions of entire muscle masses.
- **Fire** manifests as the metabolic heat of the body and its digestive processes, its mental digestion and its temperature. Biological Fire is to the organism what the sun is to the solar system, the original source of energy.

- **Water** as a biological manifestation provides the liquid parts of the body's juices. It manifests in mucous, plasma, synovial fluid, in tears, stomach acid and saliva.
- **Earth** manifests in the substance of our bodies, the structure that all the fluids, metabolism, movement and spaces exist within. It is in the bones and teeth, the eyes and ears, the hair and nails, the mitochondria and cell membranes.

As seen in Chapter 2, Air, Fire, Water and Earth manifest sequentially from out of Ether, in which they are potentialities. Earth is therefore the last element to manifest, and all matter derives from it. All five elements co-exist in all matter. Matter and energy are one. Einstein wrote equations to verify this, and he conceded that the thoughts of God were what he sought to uncover in his research.

Ayurvedic physiology has four main aspects: The *Doshas* (body humours), the *Dhatus* (body tissues), the *Malas* (body wastes) and *Manas* (mind). We shall first consider the Doshas. Tridoshic theory considers the body humours, including their relationship with mind.

TRIDOSHIC THEORY

The Vedic seers formulated a system for the maintenance and restoration of health for use by their fellow mortals and called it Ayurveda. At the level of matter as living systems we are interested in the biological counterparts to the elemental energies. On the physical plane, where for the most part we live and breathe and have our being, the biological versions of the elements combine their qualities, functions and energies in pairs, to form three functional energies, humours or *Doshas*. 'Tridosha' means 'three Doshas'. The Doshas in Ayurveda assume the same importance that Yin and Yang have in the Chinese system.

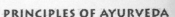

The Doshas are not 'things' to be touched or tasted, but their actions and qualities can be perceived by our senses so we know they are present when we learn what qualities to associate with them.

The elements pair off to form the Doshas thus:

Air and Ether   Combine to form the functional energy of Vata, which in Sanskrit means 'air' and also, 'wind'.

Fire and Water   Combine to form Pitta, which means 'fire'

Water and Earth   Combine to form an energy called Kapha ('water flourishes' in Sanskrit)

It is important to learn the ancient terms for these energies, because they are untranslatable in their complexity. Also, this helps avoid confusing Vata (air Dosha) with the element Air, for example.

We will examine these Doshas in relation to the functioning of the body in later sections. First, let us examine what the combining of the elements in pairs implies for the qualities of these three energies.

VATA

Vata has the attributes (both qualities and actions) of Air and Ether elements, separately and combined. Vata will sometimes manifest its Airy nature, sometimes its Etheric nature, and at times have a combined energetic effect. Predominantly, Vata is Air. Its qualities can be experienced if we think of the sight of wind-eroded landscapes, of the cooling of the skin as sweat is evaporated by a summer breeze, or of the wind created by eating a chilli con carne with lots of beans!

PITTA

Pitta has the properties (separate and combined) of Fire and Water, but is predominantly Fire. Its properties are accessible to

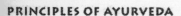

our senses as heat from the sun, as its intensity (no flame, be it ever so small, will not burn the hand that touches it) and as the light it produces. The seemingly paradoxical combination of Fire and Water can be thought of as follows: the elemental fire of a flame would consume the body, so the fire in Pitta is a liquid fire (hence the Water) and is found in such fiery substances as gastric acid and bile. Gastric acid is an extremely powerful version of hydrochloric acid and can burn its way through to the backbone of unfortunates whose gastric mucosa self-digests (as in a perforated ulcer). Bile is not quite as burning in its action, but as we recognize when we are sick, it scalds enough for us to feel the need to gargle and sip water until its effects on our throats are neutralized. It is also a bright yellow colour, and yellow, orange and red are fire colours. Also, both gastric acid and bile are transforming substances, which is a function of Fire.

KAPHA

Kapha is predominantly Water but also has the properties of Earth. Think of the stability and solidity these elements create compared to the effects of Air and Ether, think of how Kapha will be more static and heavy like a rock as compared to a gas.

AN ENERGETIC SYSTEM

Remember that Ayurveda is an energetic system and that such systems utilize the qualities of things to categorize them. Also, bringing to mind the 'as above, so below' principle, we must look at how the qualities of Air, Fire and Water as they exist 'out there' relate to 'in here', that is in our body, mind and spirit.

If it seems that I have made a subtle but profound leap from talking about elemental Air/Ether, Fire/Water and Water/Earth to air, fire and water 'out there', it is because all of these things are related (as you will, of course, have grasped). Now

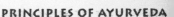

that we are talking about the gross physical plane it helps to
relate the Doshas somewhat to this level of creation, though
they are not themselves air, fire or water any more than they are
Air, Fire or Water. They are functional energies with certain
properties.

If I am belabouring this point it is because understanding the
qualities of Vata, Pitta and Kapha will assuredly enhance your
understanding of yourself, others and the whole of life. The
ability to apply this understanding gives you the choice of creating balance in yourself.

THE QUALITIES OF TRIDOSHAS

VATA	PITTA	KAPHA
Air/Ether	Fire/Water	Water/Earth
Erratic, for example wind that is changeable. The digestion may be erratic	Intense, as in the heat of a flame. Anger	Stable/Static, that is not easily changed. Not easily perturbed
Light (opposite of heavy), for example a birch tree or a small-boned person	Light (not dark), for example sunlight. Blonde to red hair	Heavy, as in the mass of mountains or big-boned or heavy-headed/sluggish
Cold, as in chilly weather and poor circulation	Hot, as in summer and body temperature	Cool, as in weather and skin temperature
Mobile, as in always in motion, activity-orientated	Spreading as in fire or a rash	Smooth, as in the texture of fats/oils Complexion
Rough(ening), as in the effect of wind erosion Hair or skin	Oily, as oil feeds fire and skin type	Soft as in the sponginess of a peat bog or a mellifluous voice
Dry, as in climate, hair, mouth	Liquid as in acids, melted solids	Moist as in marsh lands, saliva

Clear as in unclouded or clairvoyant	Sharp as in memory, a pointed nose or a spear-shaped tree	Cloudy as in skies, urine, thinking
Subtle, that is non-material, a thinker/ponderer	Sour taste and fleshy smell	
		Dense as in concentrated substance or physical build
Astringent taste		Sweet and salty tastes

HOW THE BODY WORKS: THE TRIDOSHAS AS PHYSIOLOGY

We have seen earlier how the elements relate to the structure of the body. We can now go on to how the biological energies that they combine to create relate to the body's functioning. There are three types of activity going on in the body continuously:

1 Natural functioning is maintained in cells and entire organ systems.
2 Growth, maintenance and repair of tissues (*Dhatus*, of which there are seven).
3 Excretion of wastes (*Malas*) from cells and organs.

The functioning of the body is maintained by the interaction of the three Doshas. The word 'Dosha' in Sanskrit means a fault, not as in blame but as in some flawed thing liable to malfunction at any moment.

The Doshas are (paradoxically) both essential to the body's functioning and liable to throw it out of kilter. When performing their ascribed tasks and moving on and out of the body and staying in relative balance one with the other, they are the foundation of health. If any one of them accumulates it will eventually and inevitably give rise to problems of a physical and/or mental-emotional nature. How they do this and what

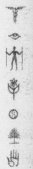

PRINCIPLES OF AYURVEDA

26   problems they can cause will be considered later on.

The Doshas respond to external causes such as beans in your diet or a rushed lifestyle. What our minds and bodies experience as a result is the increase of a Dosha (Vata in the examples given above), not the direct effect of an outside force. If the functional integrity of the body is good it will cope well with this temporary increase and eliminate it.

Vata in the body is responsible for all movement. Indeed, Vata embodies the principle of movement. Thus, sensory and motor nerve conduction is due to the presence of Vata.

Pitta in the body is responsible for metabolism, being as it is the principle of transformation from one state to another. This includes the transformation of food, air, water, from external substances to the biological substances our bodies can utilize. Thought is also metabolized (if Pitta is in a good balanced state) and integrated.

Kapha builds substance, being the principle of stability, solidity and cohesion.

PSYCHO-PHYSIOLOGICAL FUNCTIONS OF TRIDOSHAS

VATA	PITTA	KAPHA
Respiration	Digestion (the action of enzymes, acid, etc. on food)	Creation, repair and maintenance of body tissues
Swallowing (liquids and food)	Absorption (the biochemical aspects of the process)	Nutrition of the tissues
Elimination (urine, faeces, flatus and foetus)	Assimilation (the act of making what you have taken in – food or	Strength

PRINCIPLES OF AYURVEDA

	information – part of yourself)	
Movement (all voluntary and involuntary movement)	Vision	Stamina
Absorption (the movement of food in the digestive tract and of molecules from it into the bloodstream)	Comprehension, Appreciation, Recognition, Evaluation, Discrimination and Discernment	Calmness Immunity

We can see from the lists relating the Doshas to qualities and functions (above and page 24) that these energies have attributes that can be both the things they *are* and the things they *do*. So, Vata is light and makes things lighter, it is cold and chills things down, it may not be rough, per se, but as wind it roughens as it erodes.

The psycho-physiological functions of the Doshas seem to separate them into activity-orientated Vata, transformational Pitta, and substance-building Kapha. But this is over-simplistic. Yes, Vata has movement, but it also initiates transformation including metabolism, which is governed by Pitta. It is so easy to see Kapha as only structure and matter because of its relative density, but it is also the energy that maintains the body. It creates the physiological energy to keep the organism going, maintain it and repair it. The three Doshas are inextricably linked and must maintain a balance for health to prevail.

WHERE ARE VATA, PITTA AND KAPHA?

As biological energies that can be balanced or imbalanced, the Doshas have homes in the body parts where they will first start to increase if they are going to go out of kilter, and to where

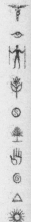

28   they must be brought back before excess can be eliminated.
They can only be directly eliminated from their main sites, their
true homes, and not from parts of the body to which they may
go walk-about when they overrun (see Chapters 4 and 5 on
imbalances and re-creating balance).

SITES OF THE DOSHAS IN THE BODY

VATA	PITTA	KAPHA
Colon (main site)	Small intestines (main site)	Stomach (main site)
Pelvic cavity	Stomach	White matter of brain
Thighs	Sweat glands	Meninges
Ears	Blood (red blood cells)	Cerebro-spinal fluid
Bones	Fascia	Saliva
Skin (organ of touch)	Eyes (organ of sight)	Sinus secretions
	Subcutaneous fat	Peri-pleural, -cardial fluid
	Skin	Gastric mucous membrane
	Liver (main organ of metabolism)	and gall bladder
		Synovial fluid
		Serum

VATA, PITTA, KAPHA AND TIME

If Vata, Pitta and Kapha are biological energies within the body
and mind which are responsible for their structure and function,
then similar forces must exist 'out there' in places, foods, plant
medicines, etc. So, at this level of creation, Vata, Pitta and Kapha
are organizing principles in the external world of matter and in
the psychic world of spirit and mind as well as in the body.

Time is movement. Chronological time is based on the movement of the earth round the sun, the diurnal rhythm of day and

PRINCIPLES OF AYURVEDA

night. Biological time is related to the biological Doshas, when the various organs are most active – activity is movement. The various stages of human life are also related to the Doshas. They are the seasons of our lives and are often referred to as such. The Tridoshas relate to all these different sorts of time.

Likewise, psychological time is the movement of emotions and feelings and, of course, these too are governed by the functional energies of Vata, Pitta and Kapha.

The following diagram links the times of day presided over by each of the Doshas with the organs they are sited in and therefore when the said organs are most active. This is because *prana* (the life-force) is highest in the various organs at the times of the day indicated. However, the information presented in this diagram should be used as a guide only, as it is based on what is happening at the equinox near the equator (the location of the Indian subcontinent).

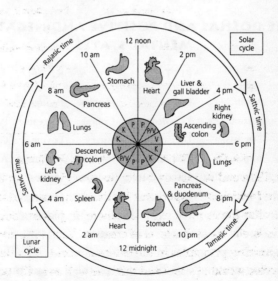

Doshic Biorhythms of the Main Organs and
Psycho-chronological Time

Looking at the diagram, we can relate health problems involving certain organs to the time of day or night. For example, gastric ulcers are more likely to perforate in the early hours, because that is when prana is most active in the stomach. Early morning and evening are when mucus collects in the bronchial system under the influence of Kapha and certain types of asthma are likely to be worse. During Pitta times hepatitis sufferers will suffer itching, while gastritis and colitis will be provoked. Similarly, degenerative arthritis and irritable bowel may make their presence felt most during Vata times.

DOSHAS AND MANAS (THE MIND)

When well balanced, the Doshas exert positive mental-emotional effects, otherwise they manifest as negative qualities, traits or attitudes.

THE DOSHAS AND POSITIVE AND NEGATIVE MENTAL STATES

VATA		PITTA		KAPHA	
Positive	*Negative*	*Positive*	*Negative*	*Positive*	*Negative*
Active	Anxious	Knowledgeable	Critical	Peaceable	Possessive
Creative	Depressed	Decisive	Angry	Loving	Greedy
Friendly	Insecure	Ambitious	Envious	Compass-	Acquisitive
Clear	Ungrounded	Discriminating	Jealous	ionate	Overly
Inspired	Restless	Logical	Irritable	Caring	attached
Flexible	Unstable		Judge-	Inclusive	
	Fearful		mental		

As the diagram on page 29 indicates, the various times of the day relate to how the Doshas affect the mind as well as the body. So if we are unbalanced in the direction of Vata, for example, then the negative emotions that relate to Vata will manifest more determinedly at Vata times – dawn and dusk. Likewise, Pitta and Kapha negative emotions will be most likely felt at midday/midnight and early morning/evening respectively. Between 4 and 8 both morning and evening are times governed by both Vata and Kapha as far as bodily functions are concerned, and also when *Sattva*, the principle of clarity and balance, is predominant in the mind. This is obviously a good time to meditate and do yoga, since these qualities enhance our inner awareness. For the remainder of daylight hours (from 8 a.m. till 4 p.m.) our minds are too rajasic (*Rajas* is the principle of dynamic energy and movement) for them to be conducive to meditation. Night hours from 8 p.m. to 4 a.m. are tamasic (*Tamas* is the principle of darkness, inertia and dullness) and again meditation will not come easily and we would be inclined to 'drop off'. Winding down after the day's activities and sleep are what those hours are for.

Stages of life have already been mentioned as a form of time governed by each of the three Doshas. Kapha governs the early years up to adolescence, gradually easing into Pitta time from early adulthood to the onset of old age, when Vata governs. It is quite easy to see the qualities of the Doshas in these life stages. The early years are years of growth (anabolism), plumpness (known as 'puppy fat'), moistness as in the dewy complexion of children and the predisposition to snuffly noses. Gradually Pitta takes over and striving ambition, drive, activity, energy and achievement are characteristic of our adult years. This is the time of 'doing'. As we move towards retirement or at least the change of pace in life that most people desire (circumstances permitting), Vata takes over as the force governing our body/mind and experience. Vata time is characterized by breakdown (catabolism) as the ageing body replaces cells less rapidly and less efficiently, dryness as the tissues dehydrate, and lightness as body mass and bone density decrease.

Seasons too have their Dosha. The relative heat of the summer sun, the bright light of sunlit days, the intense colours of summer flowers all reflect the qualities of Pitta. Pitta time includes the late spring. Winter and early spring reflect the qualities of Kapha, the time of wet and cold, of dull, heavy skies. It is a time when we find it more difficult to rise and hibernation beckons – Kapha-related qualities. Autumn is the Vata season when the temperature and climate are erratic; leaves are turning and drying out and are on the move – off the trees.

These Doshas expressed in Nature have an effect on the creatures living through the seasons. During each season the qualities it possesses build up within us and often result in imbalances that manifest at the end of the season. One good example is spring colds. Just as the weather seems to herald the arrival of spring many people succumb to colds. These are the result of the build-up of Kapha during the winter months. To get rid of such accumulated Doshas, seasonal purification is advised (see Chapter 5).

SUBDIVISIONS OF THE TRIDOSHAS

The three Doshas are subdivided according to function, area of action and (in the case of Vata, as principle of movement) direction of movement. Each Dosha has five subdivisions.

THE FIVE SUBDIVISIONS OF VATA

1 Prana
2 Udana
3 Vyana
4 Samana
5 Apana

The term *Vayu* is often used to denote Vata in combination with the names of its subdivisions.

PRANA VAYU

Prana Vayu moves in and down and is responsible for all higher sensory functions of the body including recent memory, breathing in, swallowing, central and peripheral nerve conduction, the movement of ideas and thoughts. Its area of functioning is mostly above the diaphragm, though the ascending and descending nerve tracts of the spinal cord are governed by Prana. The name 'Prana', the breath of life, is also given to the life energy, life-force or vital force known in Chinese medical philosophy as 'Chi', and is different from Prana Vayu.

UDANA VAYU

Udana Vayu functions in the same area of the body as Prana Vayu, but up and out. So, exhalation, spitting, crying, sweating, vomiting and remote memory are functions of Udana. And, as it rules the throat area, modes of self-expression like speaking out, communicating, singing, whistling, sobbing and laughing are similarly its domain. Expression of will is also the province of Udana, as exemplified by the ability to express one's beliefs, needs and desires. The balance necessary between Prana and Udana is clear. For example, breathing must be co-ordinated.

VYANA VAYU

Vyana Vayu is centred in the heart and is responsible for the movement of all circulation (blood and lymph) round the entire body and the maintenance of blood pressure. It also governs the actions of the joints.

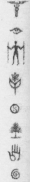

SAMANA VAYU

Samana Vayu is seated in the solar plexus and extends its effect into the stomach and the small intestine as far as the ileocaecal valve (where the small intestine becomes the colon, just below the appendix). It is therefore responsible for Vata's functions in digestion, as in the movement of enzymes and hydrochloric acid, absorption and assimilation and the mass movement of smooth muscle in peristalsis, and also in the stomach's churning of its contents.

APANA VAYU

Apana Vayu is sited in the pelvic cavity and conducts the down and out movement of flatus, faeces, foetus, urine, menstrual blood, semen, ova and the ongoing production of sperm in the male testes.

THE FIVE SUBDIVISIONS OF PITTA

1 Sadhaka
2 Alochaka
3 Pachaka
4 Ranjaka
5 Bhrajaka

Like the subdivisions of Vata, each of these is associated with different sites in the body and mind.

SADHAKA PITTA

Sadhaka Pitta's sphere of action is in the brain as the physical seat of consciousness, the mind and, mainly, the heart. Its function is thinking, processing and assimilating raw sensory input into our own thoughts and ideas. It turns sensation into perception, and processes electromagnetic energy from food to nourish the mind. Sadhaka deals with mental and emotional processing – getting to the 'heart of the matter'. It is responsible for will power and the drive to achieve in life.

ALOCHAKA PITTA

Alochaka Pitta is present in the eyes (mainly in the retina) and co-ordinates with Sadhaka to create one image from two organs of sensory input and three-dimensional vision. It is responsible for eye colour and shine. Also, Alochaka Pitta is present in the 'third eye', the pineal gland, and is responsible for spiritual vision.

PACHAKA PITTA

Pachaka Pitta is mainly located in the stomach and small intestines where it functions to digest, absorb and assimilate by its presence in enzymes and gastric acid. It is present in the liver, gall bladder and the pancreas and is also responsible for the maintenance of deep body temperature.

RANJAKA PITTA

Ranjaka Pitta resides in the liver and spleen, from where it gives colour to the skin, hair, faeces, urine and to the red blood cells. It functions to produce, maintain and ultimately destroy the population of red blood cells.

BHRAJAKA PITTA

Bhrajaka Pitta resides in the skin, is responsible for surface temperature, surface metabolism (absorption of substances through the skin including sunlight) and the same lustrousness in the skin that Alochaka Pitta imparts to healthy eyes.

THE FIVE SUBDIVISIONS OF KAPHA

1 Tarpaka
2 Bodhaka
3 Avalambaka
4 Kledaka
5 Shleshaka

TARPAKA KAPHA

Tarpaka Kapha resides in the brain and spinal chord where it lubricates, buffers and protects delicate structures. It exists in cerebro-spinal fluid. It provides the material of neurones.

BODHAKA KAPHA

Bodhaka Kapha exists in the mouth as saliva for the lubrication of chewed food, as the carrier of digestive enzymes for its initial breakdown and as the organ of taste. The six tastes in Ayurveda will be dealt with in the section on diet.

AVALAMBAKA KAPHA

Avalambaka Kapha is housed mainly in the chest as mucous and lubrication for the lungs (pleura) and the heart (pericardium).

KLEDAKA KAPHA

Kledaka Kapha exists in the stomach and intestines as the mucus lining that protects these organs from the ravaging effects of stomach acid and the mechanical damage done by the passage of rough substances through the digestive tract day after day. It breaks down particles of food so that they can be more easily reached by the digestive juices containing enzymes, etc.

Shleshaka Kapha is located in the joints where it exists as the lubricating substance known as synovial fluid. It nourishes bone.

BODY TISSUES (DHATUS) AND WASTES (MALAS)

We will now look at the other two of the four main aspects of Ayurvedic physiology: body tissues and wastes. The related concepts of *Agni* and *Ama* are included, as they are essential to appreciate how the main aspects function and inter-relate. For example, you need to know how Ayurveda regards digestion to understand how nutrients can go on to nourish the tissues.

AGNI AND AMA

Agni is the heat energy, the fire of metabolism that transforms both food and thoughts and makes them part of us. Until converted by the power of Agni they are more or less foreign to our body/mind system and if not processed thoroughly or eliminated they become toxic waste, *Ama*.

The toxic matter, Ama, is the root cause of all disease. It increases when Agni is inefficient, when it is below optimum (for reasons that will be examined later on). Ama is similar to Kapha's physical manifestations, being cold, heavy, sticky and moist. It is also malodorous. It is therefore an ideal medium for the growth of bacteria and for creating blockages.

Bodily Ama first appears in the digestive tract as a result of the poor breakdown of what is eaten. This partially digested sludge coats intestinal walls, and in this and other ways, blocks absorption. Some of it enters the circulation and, by narrowing blood vessel, is easily equated with such things as cholesterol deposits. At later stages even more insidious biochemically

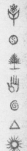

altered forms of it circulate in the body. These toxins seek homes in weakened body parts to create disease.

Likewise, the undigested experiences of life, the ones we hold on to, cannot understand and will not learn from can create mental Ama, which is even more tenacious and toxic than unprocessed food. The more subtle a substance, the more levels of body/mind it can penetrate. Mental Ama will throw damp dross on the fires of digestion and dowse Agni. This in turn will ensure that our physical digestion and metabolism are impaired, which creates more Ama, so a vicious circle is established.

The traditional view of Pitta as the container of Agni reflects their intimate connection. Agni is the heat energy within Pitta which performs the digestive function; they therefore share some characteristics. They are both hot and sharp and light, but whereas Pitta is oily and liquid, Agni is dry and subtle. It is responsible for changing the state of ingested substances into what our body/mind can use.

There are 13 Agnis that transform raw substances (food or thoughts) that are presented to them. They are:

1   Jathar Agni, the gastric fire.
2–6   Bhutagni – one to convert each of the elements (Ether, Air, Fire, Water and Earth) existing in material substances into their biologically-acceptable counterparts.
7–13   Dhatu Agnis – each associated with one of the body tissues and partly responsible for its proper formation.

It is also necessary to mention that some authorities add to this list:

- The five Pitta Agnis (one for each of the subdoshas)
- Two Pilu and Pithar cellular Agnis, which work at the atomic and chromosomal level and beyond, converting the subtlest forms of nutritive substances into consciousness. This is why what we eat determines who we are.
- One Brahmagni, the fire of awareness which transforms.

The subtler forms of Agni are more easily understood if you keep in mind the transforming power of fire. It also pays to remember to give total attention to the food you are eating, because it affects your consciousness. Do not eat when you are upset or angry; do not eat while watching television or reading a newspaper; these things are absorbed and digested along with the food and affect the functioning of Agni.

As you will see in later sections, the strength of Agni is a major factor in disease-formation. To maintain health requires well functioning Agni which affects life span, immunity, strength and energy level, colour and lustre of skin, correct conditions in the gut for friendly flora to thrive and, therefore, optimum digestion, absorption and assimilation.

SUBTLE DIGESTION AND TASTE

There are six tastes in Ayurveda: sweet, sour, salty, pungent, bitter and astringent. Each one is associated with a pair of the great elements and its effects, therefore, are due to the qualities of its constituent elements.

1 The **sweet** taste gives energy and increases body bulk. It increases blood sugar levels, slows metabolism and makes one heavy and sleepy after meals. Its association with Kapha Dosha and the elements of Water and Earth is easily recognized.

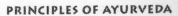

2 **Sour** has the elements of Earth and Fire. It increases digestive enzymes, which, of course, are Pitta substances. It increases salivation (think of biting into a lemon and see what happens). The Earth increases the thickness of mucus secretions in the respiratory tract.

3 The **salty** taste consists of the elements Fire and Water. The salty taste increases salivation and the flow of gastric juices, thereby improving digestion, absorption and assimilation. It eases gases and spasm in the colon.

4 **Pungent** holds the elements of Air and Fire; Air feeds Fire and produces the heat that is characteristic of this taste. There is no problem understanding that it improves circulation. Agni is stimulated in the digestive tract, and there digestion is assisted.

5 **Bitter** contains the Ether and Air elements and is therefore cooling in its action. It reduces sugar levels in the blood and lowers fevers. It enhances all the other tastes.

6 The last taste, **astringent**, is comprised of Earth and Air. It reduces bleeding time, tones tissues and dries out the food mass to be eliminated as faeces.

You will encounter the word *Rasa* in subsequent sections. It has numerous meanings, many of which are linked at deeper levels of understanding. Many 'Eureka!'-type experiences are likely to be part of your travels with Ayurveda as you integrate it into your life as lifestyle, diet, meditative practices or self-healing techniques.

Rasa is used here to refer to the initial taste something has when your taste buds relay information to the brain via sensory nerves and you perceive the flavour of something, which is a combination of all the tastes it stimulates. This taste correlates with the effects given above.

The delayed effect of taste is called *Virya* and means strength or potency (as in virility). At this stage in our exploration of Ayurveda it is sufficient to restrict the potencies looked at to 'hot', which increases digestive capacity, and 'cold', which reduces it. The other qualities of substances will be subsumed under these two. Three of the initial tastes have hot Viryas and three have cold ones. Can you work out which has which?

The long-term effects of substances on the body are *Vipaka*, or post-digestive taste. There are three: sweet, sour, and pungent.

RASA, VIRYA AND VIPAKA

Initial taste (Rasa)	Elements	Delayed effect (Virya)	Long-term effect (Vipaka)	Increase/Decrease in Dosha
Sweet	Earth + Water	Cold	Sweet	Decrease in Vata and Pitta, Increase in Kapha
Sour	Fire + Earth	Hot	Sour	Decrease in Vata, Increase in Pitta and Kapha
Salty	Fire + Water	Hot	Sweet	Decrease in Vata, Increase in Pitta and Kapha
Pungent	Air + Fire	Hot	Pungent	Increase in Vata and Pitta, Decrease in Kapha
Bitter	Air + Ether	Cold	Pungent	Increase in Vata, Decrease in Pitta and Kapha
Astringent	Air + Earth	Cold	Pungent	Increase in Vata, Decrease in Pitta and Kapha

Finally with regard to 'taste' there is the Ayurvedic concept of *Prabhava*, which is the idiosyncratic effect of some substances. Some things just don't follow the rules indicated by the initial taste, delayed effect and the post-digestive (long-term) taste or effect. Their ultimate effect on the mind/body is variable depending on the person's constitution and imbalance, and can only be learned by experience.

STAGES OF SUBTLE DIGESTION

In Ayurveda the movement of food through the digestive system is described as phases governed by each of the six tastes. So, the sweet taste is stage one of digestion, starting in the mouth and stomach (first hour and a half). It is governed by Kapha and it releases sweetness (Earth and Water) into the bloodstream.

Stage two is sour and lasts through the remaining 90 minutes or so in the stomach. Acidity is released into the bloodstream. This and stages three and four (salty and pungent) are governed by Pitta.

The final two stages (five and six) of subtle digestion, bitter and astringent, are governed by Vata. Bitter enzymes characterize the fifth stage; in the colon the astringent taste binds the content to form stools (Air, being drying, enables the reabsorption of much water and the Earth brings solidity to the contents).

THE SEVEN TISSUES

Unlike the Doshas and subdoshas, the tissues (*Dhatus*) have a specific and sequential order of appearance. Each of the seven Dhatus receives sustenance from and is stimulated to grow by the Dhatu prior to it in this chain. That is, each is a prerequisite of the subsequent tissues.

Also produced at each stage are secondary tissues (*Upadhatus*), which differ from the primary tissues in that they are physiologically dead ends. They do not contribute to the formation of the next tissue in line, though they are useful to the organism while they are around.

The third category of substances produced in tissue manufacture is waste (*Malas*). No manufacturing plant produces only high-quality finished end-products. All have some by-products, including wastes. However, the more efficient the plant, the less waste and the more top quality product are produced. Likewise here in the Dhatu factory: when each of the seven Dhatu Agnis is working efficiently, healthy tissue and secondary tissue production is optimal and waste is minimal. There is a relationship between Doshas and Dhatus.

The Doshas are responsible for the formation of the Dhatus. Kapha Dosha is responsible for all but two of the seven Dhatus, as Kapha is physiologically the one associated with growth, maintenance and repair. However, Pitta is responsible for blood (*Rakta*), and Vata for bone (*Asthi*). The seven Dhatus and associated by-products are listed below.

THE DHATU SYSTEM

DHATU	SITE	FUNCTION	UPADHATU	MALA
Rasa Lymph/ Plasma	Entire body	Nourishment body and mind; life's juice	Breast milk and menstrual flow	Physical Kapha – phlegm, mucus
Rakta Red blood cells	Blood	Invigoration, body and mind	Blood vessels, tendons	Physical Pitta – bile
Mamsa Muscle	Skeletal and visceral muscle	Plastering skeleton, protects, contains	Ligaments and skin	Ear wax, navel lint, snot and smegma

Meda Fat	Adipose tissue in limbs and torso	Lubrication body, voice. Feeling loved	Omentum	Sweat (the greasy part of it)
Asthi Bone	Bones, especially growing ends	Support, strong foundations to body, and security	Teeth	Nails, body and head hair
Majja Marrow and nerve tissue	Marrow, nerve tissue including brain and spinal cord	Filling, of bone and nerve channels. Also sense of fullness	Sclerotic fluid in eyes (some say head hair)	Tears and secretions from ducts
Shukra Reproductive fluids	Reproductive tissues	Procreation and creativity	None	None

The Dhatus are formed sequentially over a period of approximately 35 days. The first, Rasa, is formed within five days; each subsequent tissue takes a further five days. This must be taken into consideration in the treatment of health imbalances, as medicines such as herbs or dietary changes will inevitably take time to have an effect on the various tissues.

The process of tissue formation is as follows. Until the food you eat is absorbed from the stomach or duodenum into the blood and lymph, it is not part of you. Think of a child swallowing a bead. Assuming it does not lodge anywhere, it passes through and out.

What is absorbed is called nutrient chyle or *Ahara Rasa*. This is the raw material, which is 'cooked' by *Rasa Dhatu Agni* and turned into mature Rasa tissue, the secondary tissues (breast milk and menstrual fluid in females), and waste. It also produces a refined form of the raw material which goes on to be the stuff that is transformed into red blood cells (Rakta), secondary tissues (blood vessels and tendons), and waste. This goes on down the line.

If a prior tissue is substandard or if a tissue's Agni is deranged, then obviously that tissue will not be well formed. There are several ways that Dhatu formation can be negatively affected. Inherited tissue weakness as well as that incurred by faulty living (including a poor diet) are among them.

Other causative factors include the level of Dhatu Agni. If this is too high for a particular tissue then it will consume by heat the tissue it is attempting to process; tissue and all by-products will be burned up. If the Agni is too low it cannot process the raw material for that Dhatu. This results in excess of the Dosha that creates that tissue. For example, low Rasa Dhatu Agni will result in excess Kapha conditions, and low Asthi Dhatu Agni leads to excess Vata conditions.

The translations of the Sanskrit names of the Dhatus incline us to think of them as less than they are. Rasa is more than just the substance of lymph, and Rakta is more than red blood cells. These Sanskrit terms are meant to include all the enzymes, hormones and metabolic pathways in the formation of particular tissues.

Traditionally, the Vedic texts talk about three ways a tissue may be involved in the creation of the next in line. These are:

1   'Seeding', when one tissue sows the seeds for the next (used to describe the less apparent links between muscle and fat, for example).
2   'Irrigation', which is a connection like water feeding a field of crops through channels. Rakta demonstrates this as it flows through the blood vessels and carries the required nutrients for the formation of *Mamsa* (muscle).
3   'Direct conversion' covers such obvious examples as the nutrient plasma containing all the necessary substances for the formation of red blood cells.

OJAS

Ojas is the ultimate product in the formation of the seven Dhatus. If Ama is toxic and anti-health, anti-life, Ojas is its antithesis.

Ojas is the super-refined essence of Shukra; it is what our immunity, our entire health depends upon. Good reproductive tissue formation brings the life-sustaining subtle substance, Ojas. Ojas feeds back into the cycle of tissue formation and, with the breath of life (Prana) and the essence of fire (Tejas), acts upon the digestive process through the biological energies (the Doshas) to produce the tissues.

SROTAS, OR CHANNELS OF FLOW

The body has many systems of channels, known in Ayurveda as *Srotas*, through which it directs nutrients in and around and wastes out. Some of these channels of flow are large and physical, like the digestive tract, and others are subtle, like that through which mind flows.

When things are going well and health prevails, the channels are open and flow moves along at exactly the right pace.

However, inevitably things can go awry. There may be excessive or deficient flow, there may be blockages to impede it, or it may deviate from its correct course (for example, haemorrhaging blood is definitely flowing the wrong way).

In our Western culture it is socially unacceptable to give vent to certain natural urges like yawning and belching at certain times. If there is repeated or prolonged suppression of these, the Srotas involved may become functionally damaged (see Chapter 4).

There is one Srotas for each of the seven Dhatus: one for the functions of mind like thinking, communication and feeling; three to deal with the intake of nutrients, and three to deal with elimination. Women have an additional two Strotas: one for the menstrual flow and the other for the flow of breastmilk.

1   Prana (Air and breath of life). Respiratory system – deals
    with breathing and communication, including that with
    our higher Self.
2   Water regulatory system – lubrication, electrolyte
    balance. Includes kidneys and pancreas.
3   Digestive system – absorption of ingested nutrients,
    gastro-intestinal tract from mouth to start of large
    intestine.

THE THREE CHANNELS OF FLOW OUT OF THE BODY

1   Urinary system – excretion of wastes via kidneys
    and bladder. Also deals with electrolyte balance and
    regulating blood pressure.
2   Faecal matter elimination system – from the start of the
    large intestine to the anus. Also responsible for the
    absorption of minerals from the colon.
3   Sweat system – production and elimination of sweat via
    the sweat glands. Deals with water balance, liquid waste
    removal, body temperature and lubrication of skin.

THE MALAS

Malas are the last of the four main aspects of Ayurvedic physiology.

The three waste products (Malas) of the body are those that
the three channels of flow out of the body deal with. Though
they must ultimately be eliminated, urine, faeces and sweat
perform necessary functions while in the body.

Urine plays a part in electrolyte and water balance in the
body.

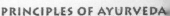

Faeces give support without which the colon would collapse in on itself. Constipation is, of course, unpleasant and produces bad breath and a feeling of malaise in the short term. If it continues over weeks and months it results in Ama and disease. However, diarrhoea brings about death in a much speedier and more certain way. The body cannot tolerate more than a few days of loss of its vital water.

Sweat moistens and lubricates the skin and helps to regulate body temperature.

The Malas are used in Ayurvedic diagnosis. For example, stools that sink, are sticky and foul-smelling indicate the presence of Ama.

PRAKRUTI: YOUR INDIVIDUAL CONSTITUTION

In Ayurveda one of the most important functions is to determine the constitution one was born with. This is a prerequisite for treating full-blown disease, redressing imbalances of the body and mind, for lifestyle and dietary counselling. All of these beg the question of what we are attempting to achieve and how we will recognize it when we attain it. We are aiming to balance ourselves (and our clients, if we are practitioners) within the limitations of the particular constitution we have to work with. Knowing your Prakruti gives you knowledge of your tendencies to react in certain ways to some foods, people, climates, events, places and epidemics. Your Prakruti is your individualized set of physical and mental proclivities.

You will have noticed that Prakruti is the same name as is given to the active, creative aspect of the universal One, which is also known as the Mother of Creation. Well, that's what your constitution is, responsible for creating you as you are as you start on your journey through this lifetime. Honestly acknowledging your true nature (at least to yourself) is the best medicine, curative and preventative that you can have. This allows you to give up that most pointless of emotions, guilt. Instead of 'why do I do, think, say, feel such and such?' or 'Why do I have flatulence, a heavy feeling in the gut or acid indigestion every time I eat a curry (and I love it so)?', self-knowledge allows you to assess realistically your psychophysical constitution. You can't change your innate constitution but you can take responsibility for changing your diet, lifestyle, etc. to create better balance.

In Chapter 3 we explored the Tridoshas, the three biological energies Vata, Pitta and Kapha that have the combined energies and qualities of the five great elements (Ether, Air, Fire, Water and Earth). The concept of constitution in Ayurveda brings together the three Doshas in a unique way for each individual. The constitution is the specific combination of Vata, Pitta and Kapha which an individual is born with. Not only that, but within each person the Doshas express themselves in a unique selection of their qualities. These qualities can appear in many guises.

The Vata qualities in one person may be different from those another exhibits. Since Vata has the combined energies of Air and Ether elements, some of a Vata person's attributes will reflect Airiness and others the Etheric qualities. One person may manifest the dry, rough and light qualities of Vata, having dry skin, a rough voice and light bones. Then again, the same qualities might show up as rough, dry hair and a very skinny, under-developed body. Another person may have completely different qualities such as erratic digestion, a subtle, philosophical turn of mind and a tendency to see the darker side of life. Consider the possible permutations of the qualities of the Doshas and of the elements that combine to form them, think of the variety of ways the qualities can be expressed, and remember that all three biological humours must be represented in every human being.

As a result of the Doshic balance in each parent at conception, the child's constitution is genetically determined.

However, the mother's diet and lifestyle during the pregnancy and all perinatal events (interventions like caesareans, inductions) will fine-tune the baby's inborn nature. Once set, our Prakruti can henceforward only be worked with to keep us emotionally, physically, mentally and spiritually healthy. The potential strengths and weaknesses are always there; being conscious of them means the difference between feeling a victim (someone things are done to) and taking responsibility for encouraging our inner strengths and minimizing our weaknesses.

THE SEVEN CONSTITUTIONAL TYPES

In Ayurveda there are seven main constitutional types: three in which one Dosha predominates, three which reflect a strong blend of two Doshas, and one in which the three Doshas exert as near as dammit equal influence on the constitution. So, you might be a person in whom either Vata, Pitta or Kapha is expressed to a far greater extent than the other two Doshas, you could be someone in whom either Vata/Pitta, Pitta/Kapha, or Vata/Kapha holds sway, or you could be one of the smaller group whose genetic and perinatal heritage has produced a Vata/Pitta/Kapha individual.

This constitutional type may sound invitingly interesting, but it has its problems. Being born with one or two Doshas predominant means that when one goes out of kilter (usually by increasing; this will be discussed in Chapter 5), the other Dosha(s) can be increased, which will usually decrease the problem humour. The saying 'nature abhors a vacuum' is true. The Doshas see-saw to maintain a balance. Treatment which therapeutically increases one will automatically bring about a reduction in the one that is vitiated. However, there is little to play around with in the case of Tridoshic constitutions that are awry! It is difficult to bring Vata/Pitta/Kapha individuals back into balance because an increase in one Dosha will require treatments that may throw at least one of the others out of kilter.

Being born with a certain Prakruti is quite different from maintaining that balance. Therefore, having a basic constitution that is Vata/Pitta/Kapha is no guarantee of health, longevity or a scintillating personality!

MENTAL CONSTITUTION: MANAS PRAKRUTI

The qualities of the Doshas are clearly reflected in both body and mind, and though often an individual's physical and mental constitutional type is the same, many people have mental and physical characteristics that reflect different Doshas. If, for example, your constitution is assessed as Vata/Pitta you may exhibit a mixture of mental and emotional traits indicating that Vata and Pitta reign jointly and, therefore, that your Manas Prakruti is Vata/Pitta. You may also have many physical features that signify either Vata or Pitta. However, it may also be the case that the majority of your physical characteristics indicate the predominance of Vata, while your mental and emotional attributes are definitely indicative of Pitta. You still are assessed as having a Vata/Pitta constitution, but the balance is very different. This will have implications for how you will tend to react to foods, people, places and situations.

Mind is obviously subtler than the body, more liable to change and not exclusively located in a specific time and place. For example, in Sankhya philosophy it precedes the manifestation of physical form and senses, while in other theories it permeates both the physical and subtle bodies. There is ample evidence that mind is diffuse and present in all body cells and that the brain is more of a receiving and broadcasting station than the seat of mind.

In previous sections I have referred to the Gunas, or attributes, of Nature (Prakruti) which are Sattva, Rajas and Tamas. In Sankhya philosophy these are seen as being potentialities in Mother Nature that come into existence as qualities of Ahamkara (the 'I-maker'). They jointly create the senses, sense organs, organs of action, the subtle and dense elements, and individual, discursive mind (as discussed in Chapter 2).

These Gunas are used in the Vedic tradition to describe states of being that reflect the spiritual aspect of the individual more than the psychological, mental-emotional aspect indicated by the Vata, Pitta, or Kapha analysis. Using Sattva, Rajas and Tamas to describe the spiritual–mental balance of a person adds another dimension to the idea of a basic constitution.

To recap, Sattva is the principle of clarity, awareness, truth and purity. It enables the individual to perceive the reality of existence with fewer ego distortions. Rajas is the principle of movement, activity and kinetic energy. It allows distractions generated by the external world, ambition and power seeking and gives the upper hand to emotions like anger and jealousy. Tamas is potential energy, the principle of inertia, and powers obstructions, resistance and dullness.

Though Sattva is the true nature of (higher) mind, Rajas and Tamas exert the necessary influence for survival in a material and materialistic world. Properly directed goal-seeking behaviour and self-defence in a life-threatening situation, or being grounded rather than a 'space-cadet' (as Dr Vasant Lad would say), are useful on occasion.

There is no direct correspondence between Sattva/Rajas/Tamas and Vata/Pitta/Kapha, so theoretically you could be a Sattvic Vata, Pitta or Kapha person. However, the journey towards Sattva could be more difficult for someone with a predominantly Kapha (heavy and dense) mind than for the

Vata (light and subtle) individual. But, as Dr Robert Svoboda would say, 'it depends'!

PRAKRUTI PORTRAITS

Although it is in the nature of things that no one can be entirely of one Dosha (because everything is made up of all five elements), it is useful to have a picture of the embodiments of Vata, Pitta and Kapha constitutions. To this end, what follows are 'sketches' of the main constitutional types. I hope that fleshing out the qualities and actions of the Doshas, personifying them, will make it easier for you to see yourself and others in these terms. Remember that these descriptions are stereotypes, and that everyone will have some of the mental and physical attributes of each of the three Doshas.

THE VATA PERSON

The Vata individual is either noticeably taller or shorter than average. This is because Vata promotes extremes. The skeletal structure is fine and light and the musculature naturally underdeveloped due to the light quality of Vata. The Vata person has dark, rather coarse hair, dark eyes (even the sclera of the eyes), uneven teeth of a darker shade of pale, dark blemishes, moles or birthmarks and skin that tans (darkens) easily!

The Vata person has a sensitive nervous system and tends towards philosophizing about life. Both of these latter attributes reflect the subtle quality of the elements Air and Ether. A congenital worrier with anxiety as a frequent companion, she often sees the darker side of things.

Vata exhibits the quality 'cold', and so it is with the Vata person. She often has cold hands and feet, usually feels the cold and prefers warm rooms and climates.

Due to the changeable nature of Vata as air and wind, many aspects of the Vata individual have a tendency towards being erratic. For example, the digestion sometimes functions well and sometimes creates problems like flatulence, gurgling gut, poor absorption. An outgoing individual may rather suddenly feel like withdrawing from social interactions. 'Changeability' may manifest in periods of active recall of dreams interspersed with times when none are remembered. Stamina is not consistent and periods of frenetic activity are often punctuated by those when energy seems very low.

The Vata person is creative and often thinks well when flying by the seat of her pants!

Obviously, not even people with very strongly Vata constitutions are going to exhibit all of these characteristics and traits, but they are common and typical of the type.

THE PITTA PERSON

The Pitta individual brings into being the light, brightness, intensity and heat of Fire. She has fair skin that tends to burn easily and blue-grey, pale blue, green or hazel eyes that tend towards light sensitivity. Sandy coloured freckles and strawberry birthmarks are typical, as is fair, blonde or titian hair.

The Pitta individual has an intense, intelligent gaze and an organizing, controlling and synthesizing intellect. Pitta makes a good executive, someone who gets the Vata creativity translated into action. This is the person who throws off winter woollens in a warm room, who quite likes the light of the summer sun but not too much of its heat, and whose glowing skin reflects some of its lustre.

Pitta has good digestion (the fires of digestion burn brightly) and physical and mental stamina. The Pitta person is of medium height, has a medium frame and good musculature.

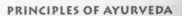

The emotions that most typify Pitta are the hot fiery ones like anger, jealousy and (at an extreme of imbalance) hatred. I had a client who decided to become vegetarian and from that day on continually told me that he hated meat eaters. He would laugh and say that he knew it sounded odd, but he did! This response reflects the emotional intensity of the Pitta nature.

THE KAPHA PERSON

The stereotypical Kapha person is large, bulky, slow moving and easy going. She is slow to anger but once aroused to it is an implacable enemy. Kapha holds on to things like this because it is created from the elements Earth and Water, the most stable and solid of the elements, and is thus not going to move location or change opinion easily.

Kapha loves to sit and, preferably, eat. She has soft, pale, cool skin, large, dewy eyes and a good head of thick hair. Generally, Kapha is cooler than Pitta but not so cold as Vata, and her sensitivity is less related to her nervous and digestive systems and more to her emotional nature. The emotions that predominate when Kapha is out of kilter are the holding-on and gathering-to-us kind, like possessiveness, greed and acquisitiveness. However, on the positive side she is calm, compassionate and loving. Kapha is good at calming down heated situations and makes for an office manager who 'oils the wheels'.

As stated earlier, someone whose constitution is of the duo-Doshic variety (whichever two are involved) will have some of the attributes of each of their constituent elements (two for each Dosha). Considering how many ways each attribute can be expressed, the possible permutations of physical, mental and emotional characteristics are legion. Nature has no difficulty producing unique individuals.

ASSESSING YOUR CONSTITUTION

There are various methods of assessing Prakruti. A highly skilled Ayurvedic physician can read it in the pulses (we will take a brief look at pulse diagnosis in Chapter 6). At this stage, by far the most reliable method of self-assessment is to look at your fixed physical attributes like your skeletal frame, your weight, the colour of your hair and eyes and so on. These, together with longstanding emotional and behavioural patterns and disease tendencies, will produce a reliable measure of your constitution.

At the end of this chapter there is a questionnaire to use in making your self-assessment. Many of us are prone to self-deception and you may be tempted to answer according to how you would like to be or feel. Please, strengthen your will and resist! If it is not an accurate portrayal of your constitution, no amount of wishful thinking will make it so, and indeed will only serve to obscure your individual reality and make it harder to find a healthy balance. Knowing how you are, fundamentally, will enable you to implement changes that can have a profound effect on your physical and emotional health and on your relationships.

ON USING THE QUESTIONNAIRE

The best way to do the following questionnaire is to enlist the help of someone who has known you for a long time. Someone like a family member who has watched your physical transformation as you grew up and has known you through the various stages of development as your mind and emotions took shape. Someone who can help you distinguish 'you' from your imbalances.

For this reason it is *very important* that you score these items according to how you have been for most of your life and/or

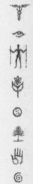

when more balanced, more 'yourself'. It is a word picture of your 'self' we are aiming to elicit, not a picture of your imbalances or dis-ease. Not all of us have recourse to old friends and family; we must do what we can, this is a counsel of perfection.

AYURVEDIC BODY/MIND CONSTITUTION (PRAKRUTI) QUESTIONNAIRE

When filling in this questionnaire:

- If possible, enlist a helper who has known you well for some time (like a family member).
- For each characteristic listed in the left-hand column, mark with an 'A' the Vata, Pitta or Kapha description that *best* matches you (not all the words in any one description will apply), as you have been *for most of your life*.
- If you and your helper do not agree on which applies most to you, leave that whole constitutional characteristic out (do not score that one at all) and go on to the next.
- If more than one description of a specific characteristic seems *equally* applicable to you, put an 'A' at each.
- Mark with a 'B' any description that seems to apply only *slightly less* than your 'A' choice.

	VATA	PITTA	KAPHA
PHYSICAL CHARACTERISTICS			
Skeletal Structure	Light frame, small boned	Medium frame and bones	Large frame and bones
Musculature	Underdeveloped, tendons quite visible	Rather athletic, well developed	Bulky, fleshy
Weight	Lightweight	Medium for height	Tends to overweight

Height	Extremes: tall and lanky or short and petite	Medium, average	Tall or short but proportionately sturdy
Colouring/ Complexion	Darkish skin or tans easily	Fair skin tones, freckles, burns easily	Pale, like alabaster, tans slowly
Skin Texture	Dry and rough, cracks in cold/ dry conditions	Soft, fine and moist, may be oily	Thick, soft and smooth, moist or oily
Iris Colour	Grey, violet, dark brown	Light blue, green, hazel, electric blue	Milk chocolate brown or dark blue
Eyes	Small, dull, eye whites – darkish	Medium, bright, prone to redness	Large, lustrous, clear whites
Teeth	Uneven or gap between front teeth, receding gums	Medium sized, soft teeth prone to decay, gums bleed easily	Strong, white, even sized, large teeth, good gums
Hair	Coarse, dark brown to black, dry, curly/wavy	Fine, thin, fair to red, can go grey early	Thick, heavy, wavy, oily, shiny, mid to dark brown
Speaking Voice	Rather weak or hoarse	Penetrating, can't whisper	Low-pitched, pleasant tone

BODY FUNCTIONS

Appetite	Variable	Keen, can't miss a meal without feeling irritable or dizzy	Consistently good
Digestion	Erratic, no discernible pattern	Very good, balances desire to eat and ability to digest	Can feel that it moves through very slowly

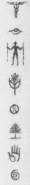

Elimination	Erratic, but more often constipated than loose, dark, gassy	Regular, loose, yellowish, at times gives a burning feeling on passing	Regular, slow, solid, bulky, mucus in faeces at times
Sex Drive	'In the head' variable, has desire but low in energy	Strong appetite, passionate, sufficient energy	Moderate to low desire, steady and strong energy
Stamina	Poor, yet dissipates energy	Medium, over-exerts competitively	Good, conserves energy unnecessarily
Pace	Everything done at high speed	Everything done at a controlled rate	Everything done slowly and deliberately
Temperature	Likes hot weather and rooms	Likes cool weather and rooms	Likes warmth but not humidity
Sleep	Difficulty getting to sleep, sporadic, wakes tired	Light but sufficient, wakens alert	Heavy, difficulty waking
Exercise	Aerobic, frequent and high energy expenditure	Competitive, balances amount with energy available	Gentle walking in countryside infrequently

MIND AND EMOTIONS

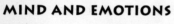

Learning	Fast learner even if only superficial interest	Has to be really interested, then can learn easily	Slow to learn but at a steady pace
Memory	Short-term recall good, long-term variable, tends to forget quickly	If interested, integrates material and retains what learned, sharp recall	Excellent long-term memory, tends to hold on to thoughts and emotions

Beliefs	Changeable	Strongly held, acts according to beliefs	Consistent, unwavering, difficult to change
Lifestyle	Spontaneous, erratic	Busy and organized	Static and repetitive
Predominant Emotion	Anxiety, fear, insecurity	Anger, irritability, judgementalism, (self-)criticism	Possessiveness, acquisitiveness and greed
Dreams	Nightmares, being chased, running, flying, fear-filled, much movement, variable recall	Violence, fire, passion, also transformation from one thing or state into another, exchange of information, money or anything and sharp recall	Romantic events, water – river, sea, swimming also mundane about everyday events, often unmemorable
Work/Project Preferences	Creative thinker, likes 'ideas' stage, a planner	Putting plans into action, making things happen, an executive	Peace-making, keeping things running well, an office manager
TOTAL 'A's	Vata	Pitta	Kapha
TOTAL 'B's	Vata	Pitta	Kapha

When assessing your constitution from this questionnaire:

- Add up all the 'A's in each column. The Dosha which has the highest score is your constitutional type and the next highest is your secondary type.
- If there is any doubt about which is highest, add on the 'B' scores to decide which is over all most descriptive of you.
- Remember, you can have two Doshas equally prominent in your constitution. A few people are tri-doshic.

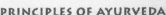

5

VIKRUTI: THE STATE OF IMBALANCE

Now that you have made an assessment of your basic constitution, the next step is to look at how you have gone out of kilter. This doesn't necessarily mean you have any symptoms of what we would generally call 'illness', but includes all the physical, psychological/emotional and spiritual distress you experience as a result of imbalance.

Usually imbalance is brought about in a general sense by an increase in one of the Doshas. The pithy Ayurvedic sutra that explains how this happens says, 'like increases like'. Whatever you eat, imbibe, look at, think about, smell or touch is taken into your 'self' either physically or as sensory perceptions, and the Doshas of these things will increase the same Doshas in you. They will do this by increasing certain of the qualities or actions that are characteristic of the Dosha in question.

If you live in a high, dry, cold area, eat raw, cold, dry, light foods like salads and frequently travel by air with your very tall, dark, nervous partner – guess which Dosha is going to be provoked? Right, Vata! All the things we take into ourselves are going to build up and affect the balance of the Doshas.

Major traumas like the loss of a partner or your home, bankruptcy or accidental injury have the effect of suddenly and severely altering the balance of the Doshas.

Often minor imbalances are caused by one-off events like getting caught in a heavy rainstorm with inadequate clothing and having to continue walking for hours in the cold. Such cases may be sufficiently redressed by spontaneous acts of caring and common sense on the part of a parent or partner who may provide warm towels, an open fire and warm, spicy foods upon our return; there may then be no repercussions.

However, our habitual diet and patterns of thought and emotion, where we live and with whom, our lifestyle (including exercise or the lack of it) and work stress levels have a cumulative effect on our doshic balance.

We are frequently oblivious to the fact that how we are living is unsuited to our type. Since our culture subscribes to the cult of the individual on the one hand but tells us we all need the same foods and lifestyle to remain healthy and the same medicines when we have the same named illness, our lack of awareness is perhaps understandable.

Knowing your Prakruti gives you this awareness, and knowing that 'like increases like' enables you to balance the Doshas in your environment (everything that is outside of the self). Everything you take in and every action you take (in other words, every interaction between you and your environment) is going to alter your doshic balance.

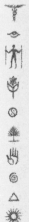

The correct progression of Vata, Pitta and Kapha is through the body performing their necessary functions (they are, after all, biological energies) and then out via the normal channels of elimination. Vata is necessary to move things around (including circulation of the blood and lymph, intestinal contents in the gut, nerve impulses in the brain and thoughts in the mind) and then it is eliminated via the colon – if all is in balance! Pitta is needed to transform ingested food and thoughts/ideas into a form we can assimilate and make part of our own body or 'body of knowledge'. 'They' become 'us'! Then Pitta is eliminated via the small intestine. Kapha lubricates the workings of vital organs like the heart and lungs (pericardial fluid and visceral and parietal pleura) and enables the smooth movement of joints (synovial fluid). It creates the substance of the body, and is then eliminated via the stomach.

Provided the Doshas are well enough balanced and the deviations that occur as a part of just being alive and interacting with the environment are small enough for the normal eliminative processes to deal with, all will be well! If you remember that your Prakruti is the individual, inborn constitution that is your unique balance of the Tridoshas, then you will realize that you are most likely to go out of balance in the direction of your predominant Dosha.

A variation on the theme of 'like increases like' is 'like attracts like'. Vata people are people in whom the characteristics, qualities and actions of Vata predominate. They are also drawn to Vata-increasing activities and substances – particularly when out of balance. A balanced Vata individual may see the point of early nights to compensate for the busy days. Memory, discrimination and determination are functioning well. However, since Vata is almost 'out-of-balance' personified, it is more often the case that the excessive physical exercise, the frenetic lifestyle and the late nights that disturb Vata are going to be part of that individual's (non) routine!

Likewise, Pitta-predominant folk may be tempted by the red meat, Mexican food, competitive sports, fiery relationships and workaholism that provokes Pitta to rise and spill over into a state of imbalance – their present Vikruti.

Kapha, being the Dosha least inclined to change, has potentially the best chance of remaining balanced (all other things being equal). However, the only thing that remains equal is the certainty that Kapha individuals are going to be attracted to the very things that will throw Kapha Dosha out of kilter – baked bananas and cream, lounging on the sofa, eating ice cream and watching soap operas.

Having provoked the dominant Dosha to the point of imbalance, it is then more difficult to treat than the other Doshas. While treatment attempts to bring about a decrease in that Dosha, the individual's own nature is tempting them in the direction of increase.

In later chapters there is information on how you can achieve balance. At present we will look at how to recognize your impending imbalances before they become recognizable diseases.

THE FIRST SIGN OF IMBALANCE: INDIGESTION

The first sign that all is not well in your internal state is indigestion, which in Ayurveda is, of course, divided into Vata, Pitta and Kapha types. Depending upon which Dosha is beginning to affect your internal balance by the 'like increases like' principle, you will start to experience one or other of these types of indigestion.

We are likely to think that indigestion is not much of a problem and that it is unrelated to real health issues. However, it represents only the first stages in the development of disease (which we will look at later in more detail), and unless resolved will progress through later stages, manifesting in very different guises and becoming more and more entrenched. Of course, often we deal with these imbalances in a similarly commonsensical way to the treatment of the cold, wet returnee suggested above. Then all will be well and our Doshas are kept in check. But when we know what we are looking for ('awareness' again), we are much more likely to do the correct things to keep us balanced or to redress minor imbalances.

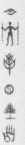

VATA INDIGESTION

When Vata starts to accumulate, its changeable, erratic nature expresses itself in variability. The digestion is fine some days and distinctly off on others, with the same foodstuffs and no recognizable differences in events. Likewise, the bowels are alternately constipated and loose, the toxic presence of Ama appears and disappears erratically and the appetite comes and goes. This is Vata indigestion. Flatulence is troublesome. There is a craving for heat including hot food and drinks. Sleep (never consistently good) is even more elusive and the predominantly Vata emotion of fear prevails.

PITTA INDIGESTION

As Pitta starts to go awry, cold food, drinks and environments are appealing. Stomach acid, heartburn and a sour taste in the mouth are present. The heat of increased Pitta liquefies the intestinal contents and produces diarrhoea. Agni (the digestive fire) is negatively affected, as any excessive liquid, hot or cold, will dowse Agni. Digestion is impaired by the increase in Pitta Dosha (a point worth taking special note of, as often there is an initial confusion between the fire of Pitta and that of Agni). As you will have correctly deduced, the hot emotion of anger will increasingly spew forth as Pitta wrests control. It is therefore worth noting how you are relating to others. If your loved ones are increasingly running for cover or taking a 'there, there' approach in conversation, which seems more and more a contest of wills ... think Pitta!

KAPHA INDIGESTION

The wet, heavy and dull qualities of Kapha ensure that the dry lightness of Agni is somewhat dowsed, and Kapha indigestion follows. What appetite remains desires light food with the astringent and bitter tastes, and the mouth waters in the way it often does before vomiting occurs – not in anticipation of some culinary delight! The heaviness is felt both in the stomach (primary home of Kapha) and in the limbs. The mind feels dull and a lack of enthusiasm for life is obvious. The desire for any exercise of body or mind is definitely not on the increase and a 'hey, who needs to work (or play) anyway!' attitude reigns.

IMBALANCES – THE ROLE OF THE MIND

Vata is going to exert a strong influence on the Manas Prakruti of even the most Kapha of individuals, as it has the same qualities of subtlety, changeability, movement and light as the mind.

The dominant culture in the West is fast, changeable and stress-inducing in everyone, including the most phlegmatic of individuals. Some people recognize the mismatch between their natures and that of the dominant culture and 'opt out'. Most of us struggle to adapt to the demands of our tribe, and in doing so bring about doshic imbalances that are mostly Vata. The pressures of modern living have profound effects on the mind.

Mind is more subtle and therefore more pervasive than the physical aspects of our being. This being so, mind plays a fundamental role in the causation of disease.

In Ayurveda the body is directed by the mind and, although there are physical causes like accidents that are outside our conscious control, many of the physical repercussions we experience are the result of a perverse and wilful determination to ignore what we know we should do. We seem to imagine that we can contravene the laws of Mother Nature and get away with it! This too has its roots in the idea, characteristic of our times, that humans are somehow above Nature and can either ignore her or command her at will.

In Ayurveda there are three forms of wilfulness:

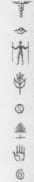

1 The Vata-related failure to remember what was the outcome of doing something – like forgetting the exhaustion you felt last week after doing a five-mile run with your athlete friend who has just asked you to train with him again.

2 The Pitta-related failure of discrimination, as in finding it impossible to decide whether or not it would be a good idea to do something you really know is a bad idea – like eating chocolate when you have started to suspect it of being connected to the occurrence of migraines!

3 The Kapha-related failure of determination, as in saying 'yes' to the very bowl of ice cream you promised yourself you would refuse after another bout of aching sinuses.

We all recognize these failures of wisdom, and perhaps even feel defensive and angry when they are pointed out as being causes of ill-health that we can avoid.

This wilfulness is one of three mental factors in disease causation. The other two factors are 1) failure to do things at the appropriate time (for example, seasonal purification, see Chapter 7) and doing things at inappropriate times, and 2) overuse, under-use and misuse of the senses and the organs of action (see Chapter 2). However, it must be clear that to indulge in these latter two, the mind must already be in the clutches of perverse wilfulness. It is therefore recognized as the fundamental cause of disease.

THE MIND LEADS, THE BODY FOLLOWS MY LEADER

Having recognized the leading role of the mind, we can now look at what the body contributes to the impending imbalance.

Mind is the subtle, manipulative and oftentimes charismatic leader, body is the naïve and easily led innocent with the brawn to create havoc.

Since our constitutional balance of the Tridoshas is thrown by the cumulative effect of the qualities of the Doshas in things and events, an improper diet and lifestyle (exerting their influence on a daily basis) are important causes of imbalance. Redressing this is dealt with in Chapter 8. A third important physical factor affecting our well-being is what traditional texts like Charaka Samhita (as mentioned in Chapter 1) refer to as the habitual suppression of natural urges.

There are 13 natural urges specified in the texts. These are the urges to:

- defecate
- urinate
- belch
- pass flatulence
- sleep
- sneeze
- yawn
- cry
- vomit
- ejaculate when aroused
- eat
- drink
- gasp for breath or pant as after vigorous exercise.

Continually suppressing any of these is going to upset the balance of the Doshas by provoking Vata (since Vata is the Dosha involved in the movement necessary to express these urges).

There are certain symptoms associated with ignoring these urges consistently and thereby aggravating Vata:

SYMPTOMS ASSOCIATED WITH
SUPPRESSING NATURAL URGES

SUPPRESSED NATURAL URGE	ASSOCIATED SYMPTOMS
Defecating	Trapped gas in abdomen, abdominal spasm, headache, constipation
Urinating	Painful urination, cystitis/urethritis, headache, can lead to kidney problems if sufficiently severe and long standing
Belching	Loss of appetite, breathlessness, hiccoughs
Passing wind	Constipation, trapped gas, urinary retention, abdominal pain
Sleeping	Light-headedness, 'spaced out' feeling, heavy eyes, tiredness, problems with concentration, anxiety
Sneezing	Headache including migraine, debility of sensory organs, stiff neck
Yawning	Central nervous system problems like tremors, numbness and fits
Crying	Runny nose, heart problems, dizziness, loss of appetite
Vomiting	Skin problems like itching and 'nettle rash', nausea, loss of appetite
Ejaculating	Pain in reproductive organs, heart pain, difficulty passing urine
Eating	Loss of appetite, dizziness, generalized weakness, weight loss
Drinking	Chest pain, dry mouth, low mood, loss of hearing
Panting	Light-headedness and fainting, heart problems

However, it is better to examine your habitual reactions to these urges (do you usually sit up in bed and read even if you know that you are very tired and could quite happily turn over and sleep?) than to try and work backwards from a list of symptoms. Symptoms are usually of a rather general nature early on in states of imbalance. If looking at your habitual patterns of behaviour illuminates consistent suppression of any of the above, you must rethink your attitude to the problem area. Many of them involve personal attitudes or habits (like sleeping when tired). Others necessitate finding socially acceptable ways to deal with the expression of these urges (a guest belching at the dinner table is not regarded as acceptable in Western society, but is a required sign of appreciation in some traditional ethnic cultures).

EXTERNAL FACTORS IN IMBALANCE

If much of our dis-ease can be attributed to our wilfulness and to what we eat and drink, indulge in and think about, some factors are beyond our control (conscious or otherwise). Also, yet other factors are choices not so easily changed for most of us, as for example what we choose for dinner. Those factors that are beyond our control or are more difficult to change include climate, season, time of day, stage of life, geographical location, the people we live and associate with and our occupation.

The climate manifests qualities of the Doshas and therefore, by the process of like increasing like, adds to any excess of that Dosha in us. Dry, cold, windy climatic conditions provoke Vata Dosha. Wet, cold, cloudy conditions increase Kapha Dosha in us. Hot conditions, particularly if also humid, increase Pitta Dosha.

Geographical location is often closely associated with climate, but also in itself has qualities of the Doshas that influence our health. Mountainous regions are high and light (the atmosphere is rarefied) and are therefore Vatagenic. Deserts are usually Pitta-provoking, though high, dry desert areas have Vata qualities in some seasons and times of day (for example when the temperature drops at night). Britain is generally rather Kapha-inducing: it is cold and damp.

The people we share our lives with influence us by the effect of their qualities on our Tridoshic balance. We know how different we can be with different individuals. People have very different opinions of us and what is characteristic of us. Some of this is projection (which is a very large proportion of our opinion about everyone we have opinions about, particularly negative ones) but there is also the effect of 'like increasing like'. Spending time with a Pitta friend is bound to increase your Pitta. If you spend a great deal of time regularly with a Pitta partner, as the years go by you may wonder about the change from the calm, benign, non-argumentative you that once inhabited your skin!

Occupation is often a reflection of our main characteristics and qualities. A serious mismatch of square pegs in round holes can lead to great unhappiness and stress-induced ill-health. It is also the case that the qualities of our work will increase the related Dosha in us. 'If you can't stand the heat, stay out of the kitchen' has literal application as well as metaphoric. Pitta chefs must be hell to work with!

The Doshas of the seasons also have important effects on our health. During each season the qualities it possesses build up within us and often result in imbalances that manifest at the end of the season of accumulation. One good example is spring colds. Just as the weather seems to herald the arrival of spring, many people succumb to colds. These are the result of the build-up of Kapha during the winter months. To get rid of such accumulated Doshas, seasonal purification is advised (see Chapter 7).

Season is an aspect of time, as are stages of life and time of day. The Doshas that predominate at each of these times accumulate and cause imbalances, sometimes during that time and sometimes just as it ends.

Ayurveda regards the joints between things (*Sandhi* points) as dangerous places and times. Whether we are referring to joints between bones, nerve synapses, times when day meets night or season meets with following season, these are times and places where things tend to be unsettled. This is partly due to the fact that the qualities, the conditions, the rules that govern each thing are in a state of flux as one ends and the next has not quite taken over. The conditions are therefore ripe for disorder and chaos to prevail. These are as related to disease as balance, order and organized functioning are to health.

It isn't the uptake of Vata, Pitta and Kapha qualities *per se* that causes problems, but whether for each individual a particular Dosha is already so high that any more reaches a level not compensated for by normal elimination of the Doshas. Any of the above factors, internal and external, can be the vehicle for upsetting the Doshic mix that is your individual healthy balance.

SAMPRAPTI – DISEASE FORMATION

Mind leads us into inappropriate behaviour like eating foods we know or suspect are not good for us, which means our digestion (mental or physical) or metabolism cannot cope well with them. This leads to the production of Ama, the toxic sludge that can then block physical or subtle pathways. Blockages mean that Vata (the Dosha responsible for movement) gets frustrated in its attempts to move in the direction it should for health to prevail. Because Vata can also move Pitta and Kapha, they too can get pushed into weak areas of mind or body

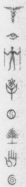

74

(*Kha-Vaigunya*, 'defective space') which are inherited or created in one's present incarnation. Disease is the ultimate result.

The Doshas can cause disease with or without Ama. The terms *Sama* and *Nirama* are used to refer to 'with Ama' and 'without Ama' respectively. It is very important when treating disease that Ama is dealt with before the excess Doshas are removed from the body. This will be explained in Chapters 7 and 8.

THE FIRST THREE STAGES OF DISEASE FORMATION

	VATA	PITTA	KAPHA
Stage One: Accumulation (*Sanchaya*). Dosha (plus or minus Ama) builds up in main site in gastro-intestinal tract. Easy to treat using Pancha Karma, which are the 'five actions' described in Chapter 7. Main problem at this stage is person's lack of will to treat imbalance	Fullness in colon, bloating, distension. Due to cold quality of Vata	Hot round umbilicus, urine/sclera yellowish, acidity. Due to liquid quality of Pitta	Heaviness in stomach, malaise, fatigue. Due to heavy quality of Kapha
Stage Two: Provocation (*Prakopa*). Still in main site but getting ready to spill out into tissues. Still able to treat using Pancha Karma	Pricking pain, chest pain and difficulty with breathing, palpitations and fullness in the abdomen. Due to cold and dry qualities of Vata	Acid indigestion, heartburn and burning in the stomach, tightness of solar plexus, excess thirst, nausea. Due to liquid and sour qualities of Pitta	Loss of appetite, heaviness in heart area and excess salivation. Due to heavy and liquid qualities of Kapha

Stage Three: Spread (*Prasara*). Doshas leave main site and enter first tissue (Rasa Dhatu) seeking a place to lodge. From now on Pancha Karma cannot be used, as it will drive Doshas deeper into tissues	Dehydration, dry skin, spasms, palpitations, tachycardia, cold hands/feet, dizziness. Due to cold, dry and light qualities of Vata	Skin rashes like acne and hives. Due to hot quality of Pitta	Oedema, coughs and colds, lymphatic congestion. Due to heavy, liquid and solid qualities of Kapha

As can be seen from this table, in the first two stages of disease formation the Doshas remain in their main sites (Vata in the colon, Pitta in the small intestine and Kapha in the stomach). This means that the treatment known as Pancha Karma can be used with impunity to remove the accumulated, provoked or spreading Doshas.

If the disease process has progressed to stages three and beyond, successful treatment becomes more difficult and Pancha Karma will not be used until other procedures have brought the wandering Doshas back home and they are ripe for elimination. Techniques known collectively as *Purva Karma* (preparatory treatments) are dealt with in Chapter 7.

It is also the case that in the first three stages the symptoms of all Vata disease is the same, likewise for all Pitta disease and all Kapha disease. One reason that this table cannot be used to accommodate all six stages of disease development is that (beginning with Stage Three and definitely from Stage Four on), each disease starts to develop its own signature which can no longer be classified as generalized Vata, Pitta or Kapha.

STAGE FOUR: DEPOSITION (STHAN SAMSRAYA)

If the first tissue (Rasa Dhatu) is strong, the overflowing Dosha will keep moving through the other tissues, seeking one weak

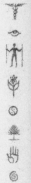

enough for it to gain entry. Degenerative changes start to occur and immunity is compromised, so infectious diseases are likely.

STAGE FIVE: MANIFESTATION (VYAKTI)

By now the Doshas are lodged in the Dhatus (tissues) and their qualities are overwhelming the Dhatus. Structural damage occurs which may persist even if the disease process is treated and halted. This is the first stage of disease according to Western diagnostic science when there are identifiable signs and symptoms.

STAGE SIX: DIFFERENTIATION (BHEDA)

The disease takes its specific form and there is no longer any diagnostic doubt about what the disease entity is. Its personality overwhelms that of the patient, who is 'not himself'. The function of the initial Dhatu and related ones is negatively affected. The person could now be differentially diagnosed as having rheumatoid or osteo- arthritis, and the different varieties of many diseases that are related to Vata, Pitta or Kapha are apparent: for example dry Vata eczema, inflamed, itchy Pitta eczema, or weeping Kapha eczema.

It is obvious from the above that it is prudent to treat imbalances as early as possible in the process of disease formation. The main problem is that we humans have the ability to ignore what we find distasteful or worrying. Having to change our lifestyle or diet is distasteful to most of us. Even having to consider that we might be vulnerable and subject to Nature's laws (God forbid, mortal) is both distasteful *and* worrying!

It is vital to note that no progression to manifestation and differentiation of diseases occurs unless the Doshas unite with the Dhatus (tissues). If the Dhatus and their associated Agnis are strong, they will resist the infiltration of the marauding Doshas and send them back to live in the digestive tract.

But an accumulated Dosha, left untreated, will cause problems with the other Doshas. Vata can push either Pitta or Kapha into imbalance. Extreme worry about job, finances and relationships, causing Vata imbalance, may be followed by an inflamed eczema of the hands as Pitta is pushed by the disturbed Vata. Likewise, Pitta and Kapha, though unable to move of their own accord, can block the free and healthy flow of Vata round and out of the body.

THERE'S NO HOLE IN THIS BUCKET, DEAR LIZA!

A good visual metaphor is sometimes used to describe the disease process. It is the image of a tap dripping into a bucket until it overflows and the spilt water spreads first round the bucket's base, then moves (as water does) to areas further afield. Eventually, the water gives life to the dried seeds of disease waiting in weak tissues and they grow and ultimately bear bitter fruits.

ASSESSING YOUR IMBALANCE

In order to make a useful assessment of your present doshic balance, your Vikruti, you can go back to the Prakruti questionnaire and complete it for how you are 'these days'. Any change in the balance of the scores for the Doshas will help pinpoint where your imbalance lies.

You can also use the table in Chapter 3 listing the qualities of the Doshas (see page 24) to assess your main problems, signs and symptoms according to the qualities they demonstrate. For example, pain *per se* is a Vata type symptom. It is transmitted via the nerves of the body, which belong to the Majja Dhatu (nerve tissue), ruled by Vata Dosha. However, the characteristics of a particular pain may relate it to imbalances in one of the other Doshas. The burning, searing, hot pain of a stomach ulcer

is rather obviously Pitta in nature, while dull, gnawing pain, like bone pain, is Kapha-related.

Other information that may help in your assessment is awareness of the external factors relevant to your imbalance. For example:

- In which season did your symptoms start and at what time of year do they now occur?
- What age were you and what stage were you at in life when they started?
- At what hour of day or night do you have most awareness of the problem? For example, noon and midnight gastric burning might indicate Pitta.
- What climatic conditions make your health problem worse or better? For example, some people's psoriasis disappears when they are on holiday in a sunny location by the sea.
- How do the geography of your environment, the people you live with or your occupation affect you? It is not a matter of 'do they?' but only 'how do they?' affect you.

What qualities does each of these areas of your life exhibit? Looking at your life now and leading up to the time when the health problem started should give you a working hypothesis about the Dosha that needs treating.

As mentioned earlier, the presence of the Doshas can go through the stages of accumulation, provocation and spread and result in imbalances even though they may not find entrance into the tissues because the Dhatus and their Agnis are strong. This means that they will not go on to the stages of what we in the West think of as 'disease'. But life with excess Doshas is not living in health, and eventually these excesses will very likely find a chink in the Dhatu armour.

The tables that follow may help you recognize the excesses of Vata, Pitta and/or Kapha that you might be living with. The first lists signs and symptoms associated with increases of each of the three Doshas. The second table gives signs and symptoms of the Doshas in each of the seven Dhatus (tissues).

SIGNS AND SYMPTOMS OF INCREASED DOSHAS

Increased Vata	Dry, rough skin with dark discolouration; emaciation; constipation, motions like sheep's droppings, flatulence; tremors, muscle twitching; tingling, numbness, dizziness and tinnitus; cracked nails, lips, nipples and anus; scanty urine and menstrual flow; desire for hot food, drinks, atmosphere and clothing; inability to slow down; pain that is radiating, fluctuating, shooting, travelling, throbbing, gripping and griping; fear of the unknown, jumping to conclusions, mood swings
Increased Pitta	Yellow tinge to the skin, whites of eyes, stool and urine; insomnia – sleep till early hours only; tired, bloodshot eyes, fainting; acidity, diarrhoea, vomiting, nausea; acne, hives and urticaria, boils and abscesses; metallic smell on breath and taste in mouth; bleeding gums; profuse menses; hypoglycaemia (low blood sugar), sugar craving, candidiasis (proliferation of the fungal organism Candida); emotionally judgmental, aggressive, perfectionist, competitive, ambitious, depressed as a result of even slight failure, perhaps suicidal, jealous, angry, impatient, irritable
Increased Kapha	Pale skin, nails, stools and urine; mucus in stools and urine; skin moist, swollen, cold; heaviness, sluggishness; water retention, oedema and swelling; loss of appetite; excessive and thick saliva; lethargy, excessive sleep and drowsiness; cold, cough, congestion and breathlessness

TRIDOSHAS IN THE SEVEN DHATUS

DHATU	DOSHA	TYPICAL SYMPTOMS AND CONDITIONS
Rasa	Vata	Skin is dry, rough, cracked, cold, hard, dark and discoloured. Dehydration.
	Pitta	Skin rashes, hives, acne, dermatitis and eczema, fever.
	Kapha	Skin is pale, cold and clammy. Lymphatic congestion and oedema, sinus and bronchial congestion, mild fever, cellulite.
Rakta	Vata	Circulation poor, cold hands and feet, blood clots, varicose veins and gout, anaemia.
	Pitta	Jaundice, cholecystitis, enlarged liver and spleen, psoriasis, eczema.
	Kapha	Thickening of blood, cholesterol, embolism, megaloblastic anaemia, high blood pressure.
Mamsa	Vata	Muscle spasm, tremors, pain, stiffness, wasting, paralysis, multiple sclerosis.
	Pitta	Inflammation of the muscles and bursitis. Ulcers, colitis.
	Kapha	Tumours composed on muscle tissue, cystic swellings in tendons, abnormal enlargement of muscle tissue.
Meda	Vata	Lack of lubrication, loose joints, dislocation of joints, low backache, lack of fat. Enlargement of spleen.
	Pitta	Boils, abscesses, urinary tract infections.
	Kapha	Enlargement and degeneration of the liver, diabetes, obesity.
Asthi	Vata	Joint pain, osteoporosis, osteoarthritis, dental cavities, brittle hair and nails.

	Pitta	Arthritis with much inflammation, rheumatism, inflammation of the bone or marrow.
	Kapha	Oedematous joint swellings and Kapha-related arthritis, bone-like tumours.
Majja	Vata	Leukaemia, anaemia, osteoporosis, paralysis and other neuromuscular problems, coma.
	Pitta	Sickle cell anaemia, multiple sclerosis, leukaemia, microcytic anaemia.
	Kapha	Tumours of the brain including the pineal gland, tumours in nerve tissue.
Shukra	Vata	Pulmonary tuberculosis, premature ejaculation, absence of sperm, depression, anxiety and other mental/emotional problems.
	Pitta	Inflammation of the prostate or ovaries, lack of sperm, sterility, menstrual haemorrhaging.
	Kapha	Enlarged prostate, stones in prostate, tumours of the testicles.

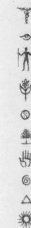

DIAGNOSIS

Practitioners of Ayurveda use various methods or tools of diagnosis which are beyond what you need to appreciate the beauty and usefulness of the Science of Life. However, assuming that you, like me, want to have a comprehensive overview, I am including descriptions of the most important diagnostic tools used by practitioners.

There are three categories of diagnostic methods: *Darshan* (observation), *Prashna* (questioning) and *Sparshan* (touch).

DARSHAN

The first method of diagnosis is Darshan (observation), which covers the visual examination of physical characteristics (for example, taking note of the client's gait, mannerisms, complexion, eye brightness), iridology (examination of the irises in the eyes), tongue diagnosis and examination of body wastes (faeces and urine more particularly).

PRASHNA

Prashna covers the practitioner's case-taking, including personal history and all the questions necessary to illuminate the problem. It also covers self-administered questionnaires like the one in Chapter 4. It is perhaps easy to see how questioning is related to diagnosis, as you will have experienced it in medical consultations of all varieties.

As far as self-diagnosis is concerned, the questionnaire is the most easily used and understood of these tools. Because any diagnostic tool is only as good as the skill of the person applying it, it is important that you rely only on such easily applied tools. It is, however, interesting and useful to have a chance to try your hand at other skills which you may decide to develop through future study. Most seasoned practitioners would rely on the confirmatory information from a combination of several of these methods.

SPARSHAN

Sparshan (touch) includes palpation (which you will have experienced if your abdomen, for example, has been examined), temperature-taking (as in feeling for variations over the body surface) and pulse-taking. Pulse-taking is the most important in this category of diagnostic methods and will be dealt with first.

PULSE

Pulse diagnosis is a skill that takes many years to hone. It can be used to confirm the assessment of Prakruti and Vikruti gauged by talking to and questioning the client. But in the hands (or rather fingertips!) of an expert, it is the most direct method of assessing these things. It is fast, cheap, accurate, non-invasive and safe. It is the coming together of the science and art of Ayurveda, technical skill and intuition.

In Ayurveda the index, middle and ring fingers acting in concert read the pulse. Pulses are never read using the thumb, as it has a pulse of its own that may confuse matters. Although

many places on the body can be palpated for a pulse, the most commonly used is the radial pulse felt at the wrist. The fingers are related to the three Doshas – Vata is read primarily by the index finger, Pitta by the middle finger and Kapha by the ring finger. Vata, Pitta and Kapha pulses can be read by all three fingers, but are most easily and strongly felt by the related finger. It is also important that, although the left side of the body is the female side and the right side is the male, both pulses are read on all persons to check for possible imbalances.

In Ayurveda there are seven levels of pulse, each providing different information:

1   Level One: Superficial Pulse. Gives information about the person's Vikruti (state of imbalance). Also can be read for six empty/hollow or semi-hollow organs. Those read on the right wrist are the colon, gallbladder and the pericardium. Those read on the left wrist are the small intestine, stomach and bladder.

2   Level Two: Manas Vikruti. Present mental and emotional state as determined by balance between Sattva, Rajas and Tamas.

3   Level Three: Information on the subdoshas.

4   Level Four: Gives information about Prana, Tejas and Ojas.

5   Level Five: Gives information about the seven Dhatus (tissues).

6   Level Six: The penultimate level is where the person's Manas Prakruti (mental constitution) can be read, and also the present state of energy in the chakra system.

7   Level Seven: The deepest pulse, where the Prakruti is read (physical constitution). This level also gives information about the six solid organs: on the right hand – lungs, liver and circulation; on the left hand – heart, spleen and kidneys.

In Ayurveda there are over 100 pulses, described by metaphor as the movement of particular animals. The three you should familiarize yourself with are those most characteristic of the three Doshas – the 'cobra' pulse of Vata, the 'frog' pulse of Pitta and the 'swan' pulse of Kapha. The immediate picture evoked by these metaphors helps us to remember the characteristic 'gait' of the pulse.

To take your own pulse, cradle one of your wrists (initially the left for women and the right for men) in the palm of the opposite hand so that the fingers of that hand can curve over the held wrist. In this position the index finger of the 'reader' hand is nearest the thumb of the hand being cradled and the ring finger is nearest the elbow. The radial pulse is found by feeling the bony bump just beneath the thumb on the held wrist, placing the three fingers along the bone and sliding them forwards on the wrist to the adjacent soft tissue. There, just enough pressure should be exerted to feel the beat of the heart reflected in the radial artery – that's the radial pulse. Because we are all anatomically unique, some people have radial arteries that are somewhat displaced. So if you don't find yours exactly as described, don't despair; you're alive, it must be there, feel around, try the other wrist!

As you take your pulse, feel its characteristic gait. Just concentrate your whole self on the quality of what you feel under all three fingers together. Is it the fast, light, slithery cobra, the bounding, stop-start of the frog, or the smooth, almost uninterrupted glide of the swan? Other descriptions of the characteristic Vata (cobra) pulse are slightly irregular, cold, feeble, narrow and empty. The Pitta (frog) pulse may also be described as hot, full, regular and moderate, while the Kapha (swan) pulse is cool, slow, steady, strong and deep.

Pulse rate is affected by many factors, but can also give information about the predominant Dosha. As a general guideline, a resting pulse of 80 to 95 beats per minute is typical of Vata, 70 to 80 beats indicates Pitta, and 50 to 60 beats is common for Kapha. Count the beats for a full minute when trying to gauge your pulse rate, and take it first thing in the morning before you eat anything.

We shall now turn our attention to Darshan, the category of diagnostic methods that deals with observation. Urine and tongue examination are the techniques we shall look at briefly.

URINE EXAMINATION

The waste products of the body are used in Ayurveda to give information about a person's state of health. Of these, urine examination is widely used by Ayurvedic physicians. You can practise your skills of observation by inspecting your own urine. The colour/turbidity, odour and acidity of urine (among other features) indicate the predominance of one or other of the Doshas. These are qualities you can easily observe for yourself.

Fresh Vata urine (that is, urine with a preponderance of Vata Dosha) is generally clear and effervescent. Pitta urine is clear and yellow. Kapha urine is turbid (cloudy white). Remember that certain foods like beetroot profoundly affect the colour of urine, and that urinating with urgency (which increases the pressure) or from a height (as in standing to urinate) will affect the effervescent quality of any urine.

If you have access to dip sticks that measure the pH of urine (the acidity/alkalinity), then you'll want to know that Vata urine is neutral, Pitta is acidic and Kapha alkaline, given a normal range of pH 4.5 to 8.2 where high is alkaline and low is acidic.

Everyone knows the smell of urine, but that is usually urine that has been standing for some time. Fresh normal urine has an aromatic ammonia odour. Vata urine has no odour except first thing in the morning. Pitta odour is strong, Kapha's is moderate. Diet can change odour, so beware of the effect of, for example, broccoli, which makes urine smell more strongly; asparagus, which gives it a horsy smell; and coffee, which adds a whiff of rodent!

There is a test you can try using a clear glass and enough urine to see how a droplet of oil spreads across its surface. Traditionally sesame oil is recommended.

Take a toothpick and dip it in the oil. From the toothpick allow one millet seed-sized drop to fall onto the surface of the urine in the glass. If the urine is Vata then the drop will immediately spread over the surface and dissipate. If the urine is Pitta, the drop will spread and produce a rainbow colour effect. If the urine is Kapha, the drop will spread very gradually.

TONGUE DIAGNOSIS

Tongue diagnosis uses the concept of one part of the body to reflect the condition of other parts (organs or systems). When a Western doctor looks at your tongue something similar is being considered. Ayurveda and other systems using tongue diagnosis apply a more detailed map of correspondences. You have probably heard of iridology (using the iris of the eye as a diagnostic map) and reflexology (using the palm of the hand or the sole of the foot for the same purpose). These tools are based on ideas similar to the microcosm and macrocosm of 'as within so without, as above so below'.

As you will now be coming to expect, tongues also are Vata, Pitta or Kapha (there are, of course, mixed type tongues also). Vata tongues are generally narrower and dry, and may reveal nervousness by trembling when stuck out of the mouth. Pitta tongues may be red, smooth, soft, shiny and clean and have a definite point at the tip. Kapha tongues are generally large and broad, rounded at the tip and moist, at times to the point of over-salivation. A diagram of a mirror-image tongue map and a few examples of what an Ayurvedic physician is looking for are given below.

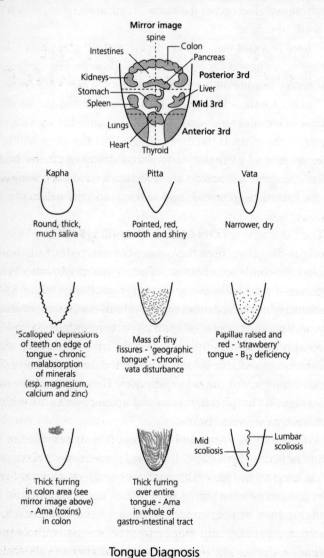

Tongue Diagnosis

7

TREATMENTS FOR RE-CREATING BALANCE

Now you are ready to look at ways to re-create the balance that constitutes health; the balance between body, mind and spirit/consciousness, and the balance within each of these aspects of being human.

The health of your body involves getting a balance between the Tridoshas that constitute your physical Prakruti. Likewise, a healthy mind will maintain a Dosha-specific balance that is peculiar to you (your Manas Prakruti), and the spiritual health you achieve will show in the balance between Sattva, Rajas and Tamas. The health of the total being depends upon the interactive dynamics of the physical, mental-emotional, and spiritual.

A balanced person is always going to manifest the qualities of his or her predominant Dosha more than those of the other Doshas. For example, a balanced Vata person will always manifest the qualities of Air and Ether elements more than those of Fire, Water or Earth; but in a positive, dynamic way. The emphasis is on 'dynamic'. Health is a process, not a fixed state.

Constantly the Doshas in us are being affected (according to the 'like increases like' principle) by our interaction with everything that constitutes our environment – the food we eat, the people we socialize and work with, the weather we tolerate or thrive in, the season that propels the year onwards and the stages of life that we are experiencing. In health these continual accretions are dealt with by natural elimination of the excess Doshas as they arise. These things we have examined already.

However, when imbalance is more than part of a fluctuation that is soon redressed, then we need to seek help. To ensure that our Doshas remain within manageable limits, we would be wise to follow dietary and lifestyle guidelines that assist in maintaining balance. These, along with simple treatments for minor imbalances, are dealt with in Chapters 8 and 9. For the present let us look at some of the treatments prescribed by Ayurvedic practitioners for their clients (finding such professional help is the subject of Chapter 10).

THE CLASSIFICATION OF TREATMENTS (CHIKITSA)

The process of disease formation in Ayurveda (*Samprapti*, dealt with in Chapter 5) involves six stages. The first three produce symptoms that are Dosha-specific rather than disease-specific. They are premonitory symptoms of what Western medical science views as disease. These stages are accumulation, provocation, and spread of the excess Doshas which, nonetheless, remain within their main sites (the colon for Vata, the small intestine for Pitta, the stomach for Kapha).

During the stage of accumulation, measures used to redress the imbalance may be limited to dietary and lifestyle advice, as dealt with in Chapter 8.

When the provocation stage is reached, substances and physical treatments that provide the qualities opposite to those manifested in the imbalance are given to rebalance the Doshas.

When the disease has reached the stage of spread, then purification in the form of Purva and Pancha Karma is required.

If the disease has progressed to such an extent that a total healing is not probable, then palliation is resorted to.

RASAYANA AND VAIJIKARANA

The Ama (toxins) which may be mixed with the Doshas must be dealt with before Purva Karma and Pancha Karma are given. After the elimination of toxins and excess Doshas come the processes known as *Rasayana* and *Vaijikarana* (rejuvenation and virilization, respectively), which can be seen from their names to be tonic and nutritive, and therefore feed the system.

SHAMANA – THE SEVEN TREATMENTS FOR PACIFYING DISEASE

These treatments are given in various situations as, for example, when the patient is too weak for more heroic methods, at extremes of debility or toxicity and also, as mentioned above, early on in the disease process when the imbalanced Doshas are still in situ.

1 Kindling Agni – sometimes Agni suddenly reduces, as in the case of diarrhoea and vomiting. If the patient is not hungry, then avoiding food for a limited time will fan the digestive fire. Mixtures of spices may be given to increase Agni.
2 Detoxifying – almost always associated with low Agni, the presence of Ama reveals itself through symptoms such as fatigue, feelings of heaviness, malaise, lack of taste, coated tongue and boredom. Again, mixtures of spices may be given.
3 Fasting – 'no solids' may be recommended in cases like flu or fever. Water, herbal preparations, fruit/vegetable juices, some light foods or a mono diet (one kind of food

only, such as kichadi – see recipe on page 172) may be given. Fasting kindles Agni but increases the light quality, so should not be continued for longer than three days for Vata, four to five days for Pitta, and possibly up to 10 days for Kapha.

4 Sunbathing – this is deemed of value even if it is seen as taking in the sun's light through the eyes and its warmth from the air through the skin while sitting or lying in the shade rather than basking directly in the sun's rays. (Remember the problem of SAD – a form of depression related to lack of light during the darker seasons – but also the problems like skin cancer/melanoma associated with the depletion of the ozone layer.)

5 Air – fresh air is recommended as treatment and, of course, prevention. Good air and good breathing are essential to tissue oxygenation. Many diseases, for example cancer, thrive in low oxygen conditions. Humans also extract the life force, Prana, through breathing (as well as from food) and so 'air' as a form of treatment can involve yogic breathing in meditation.

6 Reduction in fluid intake – this depends on the condition of the patient and the Dosha involved. Monitoring and reducing fluids may be advised in health problems such as ascites (fluid retained in the abdomen).

7 Exercise – some exercise is required in all but acute and/or debilitating conditions, and will be advised with the patient's condition in mind – from gentle walking to dynamic yoga.

SHODHANA – CLEANSING THERAPIES

These include both Purva and Pancha Karma, and can be administered after the toxins (Ama) are removed, provided the patient is strong enough, not too young, too old or debilitated. They are regarded as primary pillars in the Ayurvedic treatment repertoire.

PURVA KARMA

Purva Karma includes the preparatory treatments of oiling and sweating. The aim of oiling and sweating is to encourage the wandering Doshas to move out of the tissues in which they have taken up residence and to return to their main sites. From there they can be removed from the body using one or several of the five treatments known collectively as Pancha Karma.

Oiling can be internal or external; usually both methods are used. Most commonly, an increasing amount of ghee is added over a varying period of a couple of days to a week or so. At the same time, a kichadi diet is taken. The external oiling is in the form of massage, using oils suitable for the Dosha that is out of kilter (often sesame oil is used).

What this achieves is internal and external lubrication that eases the return to the digestive tract of the errant Dosha(s) and voiding via the relevant tract(s). A steam bath with herbal medicated steam helps perform this task by opening the pores to the previously applied oil, heating and liquefying the Ama (toxins) and moving it from the body tissues into the circulation.

PANCHA KARMA – THE FIVE MAIN CLEANSING THERAPIES

Pancha Karma is then given to remove the mobilized Doshas. Pancha Karma is also used to keep the Doshas in check before

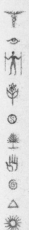

they cause problems. At the turn of the seasons, Ayurveda encourages people to have cleansing therapies to eliminate any Dosha accumulated during the season past, before it causes imbalance and before the qualities of the coming season start to impinge on the body and mind.

Not all Pancha Karma treatments are given to each individual. The practitioner decides which are appropriate, and then those are given in an accepted order. These descriptions of the five treatments follow this order.

VAMANA

Vamana is therapeutic vomiting. Elimination via the upper pathway is the main technique for getting rid of excess Kapha Dosha once it has returned to its main site, the stomach. This is clearly the most direct route from the stomach. There are many different substances that can be given to induce this emesis, including black salt, rock salt or liquorice.

Some of the presenting conditions that might benefit from Vamana therapy are coughs and colds, asthma, epilepsy, nausea and breast congestion. However, as with all Pancha Karma treatments, it is very important that a qualified practitioner examine the client first, that the requisite Purva Karma has been given and (most importantly) that the Doshas are ripe for elimination. If they are not, they will be driven deeper into the body tissues rather than voided.

VIRECHANA

Virechana is purgation therapy and it is used to eliminate excess Pitta Dosha from the small intestine. Obviously, the best exit from the small intestine is down and out via the large intestine. Purgation can be given three days after the successful completion of Vamana, if it is deemed necessary by the practitioner. Most disorders that indicate excess Pitta will benefit from Virechana – provided, of course, that the Pitta has successfully been brought back to its main home in the small intestine. Examples of such conditions include inflammatory skin diseases, worms, gout and hepatitis. Some of the substances used to induce purgation include flaxseed and psyllium seed husks, castor oil, prunes or raisins soaked in milk. It is often unnecessary to give strong cathartics to produce purgation in high Pitta conditions – Pitta is prone to promote loose bowels due to its liquid and hot properties.

BASTI

Basti means 'bladder', and is used to denote therapeutic enema as in ancient times when animal bladders were used to hold the liquid concoctions used for the enema. Vata responds well to Basti and, as Vata easily goes out of balance, enemas are frequently part of Pancha Karma.

Basti may be given three days after completion of purgation therapy. It is usual to give purgation prior to enema. There are quite a number of different liquids that may be used in this treatment, but often it is a mixture of oils such as sesame oils plus decoctions of herbs like Dashamoola ('ten roots'). Decoctions are made by boiling up the herbal substances in water for a short time (10 minutes or so) then straining off the liquid. Decoction is the method of choice for the extraction by water of the constituents of roots and other tough plant parts.

The term 'Basti' is used to cover more varied treatments than do the terms 'Vamana' or 'Virechana'. There are rectal Bastis (what we refer to as enemas), male urinary bladder and female vaginal Bastis (douches), Bastis for the eyes (surrounding the eye of the prone patient with a dough ring and filling the tiny well with oil), for the head (a sealed leather hat filled with oil round the head) and those for chronic, non-healing wounds.

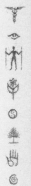

The kinds used in the Pancha Karma sequence are variations of the decoction and oil rectal enema.

NASYA

Nasya is the nasal administration of medication. It is given as a cleansing therapy in Kapha-type diseases of the head (including the brain and consciousness) and throat, such as headache, colds, chronic rhinitis, catarrh, sinusitis and epilepsy. In such cases it is usually administered as a powdered herbal snuff.

As a therapy for Vata imbalances which require nutritive substances, Nasya is given using ghee containing herbal extracts, oils or medicated milk. Problems helped by this treatment include Vata migraines, dryness of the nasal mucous membrane and negative Vata emotions such as fear, nervousness and depression.

RAKTA MOKSHA

Rakta Moksha, blood-cleansing (traditionally, blood-letting by leeches) is no longer used in the West, although there has been recent research about the beneficial medical uses of leeches.

GETTING TREATMENT

Often people book into a centre for three to five days for Pancha Karma treatment. Their food during the Purva Karma and Pancha Karma (usually kichadi) is then provided and all their basic needs are met. This has the essential benefit of allowing them to rest and relax into their therapy. It is very important that the environment is Vata-friendly during and immediately after Pancha Karma, as the necessarily light diet and the cleansing treatments that carry excess Doshas out of the body are predisposed towards vitiating Vata. A warm, relaxing, stress-free time is essential to get the most out of Pancha Karma.

PLANT MEDICINE

All traditional systems of medicine use plants. Plants were there for the earliest humans to use and, apart from touch (as when a mother rubs a fallen knee), probably constitute the oldest form of medicine.

We in the West are still finding out about 'new' herbs (the generic term for all medicinal plants) that have been used by traditional peoples all over the globe for as long as their collective memory can trace. Generally though, systems of herbal medicine use formulae that work together synergistically to redress the patient's imbalance as it is diagnosed in the terms of that system. Few of these plants would be used alone as treatment; this aspect of traditional medicine is usually ignored when a 'new' plant breaks into the world herbal repertory.

Ayurveda has a long and honourable tradition of using herbal medicine. In common with other indigenous systems, it uses some substances that are not plant in origin like bitumen and the purified and humanized forms of some metals. However, the use of these is conditional upon the law of the land in which the Science of Life is being practised. Therefore many of these substances are no longer used or, at least, no longer used where you are likely to be offered them as treatment in the West.

As we have seen already, toxins must be eliminated and the digestive fire must be optimized before any excess Doshas can be expelled. Herbs such as Trikatu (black pepper, long pepper and ginger) may be given to stimulate Agni, and mixtures containing spices such as ginger with differing proportions of ghee or honey may be given to aid in the burning up of Ama.

There are hundreds of remedies in the Ayurvedic herbal pharmacopoeia, and it would be inappropriate to include much of this material here as, in many instances, their use requires professional guidance. However, in the next chapter

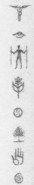

there are a few suggestions for simple household remedies.

The Ayurvedic practitioner will select appropriate remedies which are both good for the client's constitution and the condition itself. Herbal treatment will generally be given for an initial period of three to six months. If you recall the information given about how long it takes each of the tissues to be created sequentially, you will realize that it can take anything from 5 to 35 days for any substance (herbal or other) to affect the Dhatus (tissues).

After the first few months of treatment, it may be deemed appropriate to have a period of rest (lasting a few weeks). All natural remedies seem to have better results when given this way, to prevent the body from getting too used to them and (very importantly) the mind from assuming that the treatment is supposed to cure everything including Life. The same remedies may be reintroduced later, or a new mixture given.

ANUPANA

Anupana is the Sanskrit term for a carrier substance. This is another important part of Ayurvedic herbal treatment, as the right Anupana will help the medicine travel to the correct site within the body. Commonly prescribed Anupanas are honey, ghee, warm water and milk. Traditionally, herbs that are given in a powdered form (rather than as a tea, for example) are taken directly on the tongue. With the Western distaste for less pleasant tastes and the advent of capsules, it is even more important to use a suitable Anupana, as the herb's natural taste is literally encapsulated. Reread the section on taste (Rasa, see pages 39–42) and how important Rasa, Virya and Vipaka are to what your body makes of the substances you ingest.

REJUVENATION THERAPY

After treatment for Doshic imbalances or Doshas in the Dhatus (disease proper), the practitioner may recommend rejuvenation therapy including herbs such as *Ashwagandha* (particularly for Vata), *Shatavari* (Pitta) and *Pippali* (a Kapha rejuvenating herb).

ASHWAGANDHA

Ashwagandha, or Winter Cherry (*Withania somnifera*) is bitter and astringent (Rasa); heat is its energy (Virya); sweet is its post-digestive taste (Vipaka). When fresh it smells like the urine of a horse, which may not seem like much of a recommendation but think, horses are strong! It acts as a tonic, sedative and aphrodisiac for those problems that shout Vata, such as anxiety and subsequent insomnia, low libido, muscle weakness, chronic fatigue and debility in old age (amongst other complaints). It has also been used in pulmonary tuberculosis where it can heal the cavities, particularly in the apical regions of the lungs. Like the next remedy, Shatavari, it is an ingredient of Chyavan Prash, a delicious tasting jam-like preparation that is a Rasayana (rejuvenating remedy) for all three Doshas.

SHATAVARI

Shatavari (*Asparagus racemosus*) is a rejuvenating herb with a particular propensity for Pitta. Its tastes are sweet and bitter, its energy is cooling and its post-digestive taste is sweet. It is used in conditions like diarrhoea, dysentery, hyperacidity, kidney and liver inflammatory problems and as a tonic to the ovaries, the endometrial lining of the womb and the fallopian tubes. As an oestrogenic herb it is useful at the menopause in the prevention of osteoporosis. All seven Dhatus are affected by its properties. In a preparation with ghee it can help resolve non-healing wounds and ulcers.

PIPPALI

The third herb in Chyavan Prash is Pippali or Long Pepper

(*Piper longum*), which is particularly rejuvenating to Kapha. The taste that predominates is pungent, the energy is heating and the post-digestive effect is sweet. Its uses include treatment of fatty, degenerative changes of the liver, obesity, bronchial asthma, chronic dyspepsia, rheumatoid arthritis and loss of appetite.

It is important to emphasize that most herbs are used, most of the time, in combination with others so that they work synergistically – that is, they have an effect that is greater than the sum of their separate actions.

The herbs described above are examples of what might be given by an Ayurvedic practitioner. However, it must be clear by now that selection is based upon exhaustive scrutiny of the client's individual Prakruti and Vikruti, and knowledge of the combined action of a range of ingredients.

The use of plant medicine in Ayurveda adheres to the idea of there being nine causative factors in the universe: the five great elements, Cosmic Consciousness, mind, time, and direction. In the case of plants, 'time' refers to the season during which a plant matures, and 'direction' refers to where the plant grows (mango and papaya come from the South, for example).

There are Vedic deities associated with every direction and with each plant and plant part. The presiding deity is invoked near the plant, the petitioner facing East the evening before the plant is culled for medicinal use. The deity's blessing ensures that the plant's healing properties are maximized. Next morning, after meditation and bathing, the plant is picked and prepared.

MARMA CHIKITSA – TREATMENT OF VITAL POINTS

Marma points are specific places along the body surface where pressure or the insertion of needles will affect the flow of the vital energy or Prana along a complex system of subtle channels called *Nadis*. You will probably already be thinking 'acupuncture' and indeed that is what Marma treatment is, Ayurvedic acupuncture or acupressure depending upon the specific technique used to affect the Pranic flow.

Though few Ayurvedic practitioners use the ancient Bhedan Karma ('piercing-through therapy'), light-pressure Marma balancing is quite commonly used. The Adankal or finger-pressure therapists of South India still recognize over 350 Marma points which lie along the Nadis that link major organs.

Also known in Ayurveda is the concept of lethal Marma points. Among these points (of which there are over 100) are those at the temple, throat, heart, belly button and scrotum. Certainly, the Ayurvedic surgeons who in former times treated those injured in battle would have had detailed knowledge and frequent proof of the efficacy of these points. Injury at the site of these results in death. The timing depends on the relationship between the Marma point of injury and the element associated with it. Immediate death ensues if the point relates to Fire, is delayed if Water is the element involved, and occurs after the knife or other weapon of assault is removed from the wound in the case of Air.

Modern surgical procedures may affect health by interfering with the flow of subtle energy through the channels; those ancient surgeons would have been well aware of this problem too. I remember one encounter with a patient in a training session whose chronic pain and ill-health started shortly after his feet were crushed in an accident. No other injuries were sustained, and only the concept of Marmas explained the severe discomfort and dysfunction experienced at sites remote from the parts injured and not linked by the same nerve tracts.

If you are seeking treatment in the West you may be offered a general Marma balancing, starting with points on the head and shoulders, moving to the ankles and knees, then the abdominal and chest areas and finishing back at the head. Each point (or several pressed together) is held for a short duration (one and a half minutes) so that the entire treatment takes only a quarter of an hour.

GEMS – MEDICINE OF THE PLANETS

Within the Vedic system, gem therapy is associated mainly with the science of astrology or *Jyotish*. The nine main gemstones have planetary connections – included in the Vedic list of 'planets' are Ketu and Rahu. These two nodes of the moon have powerful (oftentimes dark and dire) effects on individuals during the times these nodes afflict their horoscopes, and are therefore seen as having planetary status.

Though some difference of opinion exists as to which stones placate which planets, there does exist some consensus as to the beneficial effects of the stones where a particular planet is weak in the client's horoscope. In this way gems are used for their subtle effects on the mind and emotions.

The Sun	Ruby
The Moon	Pearl
Mars	Coral
Mercury	Emerald
Jupiter	Yellow Sapphire
Venus	Diamond
Saturn	Blue Sapphire
Ketu	Cat's Eye
Rahu	Onyx

An Ayurvedic physician may use your Jyotish chart and/or your palm to make a prognosis in conjunction with diagnostic procedures, and may refer to these as an aid in deciding on your treatment.

Apart from taking account of the planetary associations, traditional Ayurveda uses gemstones as internal medicine. The gemstones are reduced via complex processes to ashes or Bhasmas (minerals). However, quite apart from other problematic issues like our acceptance of the logic of using diamonds as medicine (even if they are 'a girl's best friend'!), they are obviously very costly and difficult to produce.

Gems can, however, be used in ways that leave their substance completely intact. Gem tinctures can be produced easily, the appropriate stones can be worn, or they can be used in distant healing. All of these methods use only the inexhaustible energy of the gemstones.

The Bhasmas are used to treat physical conditions, some of which are listed in the table below.

Ruby ash	Promotes longevity; balances Vata, Pitta, Kapha; used in cases of burning sensations in the limbs; colic and constipation, boils and ulcers
Pearl ash	Promotes longevity; improves eyes and complexion; used for heart problems, palpitations, high blood pressure, breathlessness; coughs and chronic fever
Coral ash	Indigestion, constipation and lack of appetite; anaemia; jaundice; asthma; urinary disorders and obesity
Emerald ash	Hyperacidity, indigestion, nausea, vomiting, piles; acute and chronic fevers
Moonstone ash	Poor appetite, indigestion, nausea, vomiting, poisoning and food poisoning

| Diamond ash | Promotes longevity; used as a general tonic to all the tissues; treats many conditions including diabetes, anaemia, emaciation and obesity |
| Sapphire ash | All afflictions of the nervous system from nerve pains to hysteria, delusions and epilepsy |

More information about the use of gemstones and colour is given in Chapter 8.

SELF-HELP: THE DAILY BALANCING ACT

Now it is time to look at the ways in which you can care for yourself, including your *Self* (the personal Divine, the drop of the Cosmic Ocean that is you). One translation of the term 'Ayurveda' is 'Science of Everyday Life', and that name leaves us in no doubt as to what aspects of life are going to have the most pervasive and enduring effects on our well-being: Those that are part and parcel of the daily round – most especially diet and lifestyle.

No matter what we eat or how we pass our days we have, by definition, a diet and a lifestyle. Remember the second Sutra of Ayurveda, 'like increases like'? The qualities of the elements Ether, Air, Fire, Water and Earth are in everything and, according to the principle of 'like increases like', will add to our store of the relevant Dosha. By addressing what we put into our bodies and minds and how we move along the path of life on a daily basis, we can do much to restore and maintain balance.

There are other specific things that would be of great benefit if added to your life; these will be outlined in Chapter 9. These include yoga, meditation involving the chakras and mantras, and the use of herbs, gemstones and essential oils for their healing effects.

To assist you in extracting what will benefit your particular constitutional type, the following sections are arranged according to the Doshas. Remembering that such advice is aimed at the archetypal Vata, Pitta and Kapha and that no one alive can be that; blend them as you need.

LIFESTYLE

FOR THE VATA TYPE

According to the ancient wisdom, the Vata individual is a hot-house plant, so start by implementing changes gently and gradually. 'Sudden and drastic' are not generally the best ways to balance Vata, given that 'erratic, fast and mobile' are the key Vata qualities that usually need to be subdued.

Given the innate fragility of the Vata nervous system, adequate sleep is essential. Given the Road-Runner attitude of Vata, this might seem to go against the grain. Vata needs to make sure that the bed is warm (a heavier duvet, maybe even with a top blanket), inviting, and used for sleeping in – it is not for reading in, watching telly from or making telephone calls in, all of which will stimulate the Vata brain into spirals of activity just as the lights go out! To help, a sleep pattern is exactly what is required, also a design for living, a schedule. Despite the face pulling that you are now doing, Vata is calmed by regularity. Vata needs to have a prearranged time for bed and for rising and for most other daily pursuits. Do not fear that life will become boring and predictable. Setting times for the main functions in life will just take the edge off the frenzy that you live in and allow you to appreciate life as it flashes by.

To assist in the relaxation process, essential oils may be added to a warm bath before bed and also used in the bedroom. While on the subject of oils, Vata will benefit from and delight in massage, so build this in to your lifestyle. Vata is associated with the sense of touch and oil counteracts the dryness and lightness of Vata. Regular massage need not cost more than the price of a few oils, as a good friend and some enthusiasm will give you a wonderful intuitive massage, and then you can reciprocate!

Sleeping during the daytime is not usually advocated in Ayurveda as it increases Kapha. So Vata people, you should be so lucky! If you are feeling exhausted during the Vata day time (roughly 2 till 6 p.m.), take 10 minutes out. Find a warm, draught-free spot on the floor (not so comfortable that you'll sleep for hours), cover yourself with a blanket, lie in the corpse pose (flat on your back, arms and legs falling gently away from the midline of your body), and relax. If you are really tired you will probably drift off for a few precious moments. If the Vata go-go will not let you sleep, at least you will have stopped moving for a few minutes.

Because Vata's digestion too is often erratic it is sensible to eat small meals more frequently rather than a few large meals. Say, four small meals rather than the three meals that is our culture's norm.

In terms of exercise, the classic Vata type would spontaneously choose an aerobic exercise like running; something that involves a high expenditure of energy. However, to give Vata a little of what it does not have (discipline, controlled movement and energy release), a good form of exercise is yoga – more about this later. And don't exercise till you drop, just till your brow starts to perspire. You need to conserve energy.

Vata people are often talkative and enjoy socializing. However, in this too they can be rather erratic and, if out of kilter, may suddenly decide 'I want to be alone'. Much better they should take time to themselves before the need becomes urgently compelling. Scheduled times of solitude and silence in a busy life are of great benefit to Vata, though it can be hard to create the habit initially. Try writing short gaps into your diary or appointments book – and stick to them. Fill them with the silent and solitary pursuit of some gentle hobby or leisure activity. A stroll round the neighbourhood park, gardening (re-potting a plant takes little time but is very calming and satisfying), an occasional session on a sunbed and some silent, solitary meditation are all soothing to jangled Vata.

Even if the Vata imbalanced mind would rather do *anything* than succumb to meditative stillness, you can start by planning to meditate for five minutes at the same time each day (preferably before the rush of day begins – and remember, the early morning between 2 and 6 a.m. is Vata time).

So, you have written in your daily plan that these particular five minutes are for meditation. Use them to sit in the same quiet spot each day and go with your Vata mind. Just let the thoughts come and go. Don't try to stop thinking but allow the thoughts to enter, pass through and leave. If you find yourself worrying over a particular thought, just be aware of what is happening and let it go. In other words, do not spend these minutes planning dinner! Eventually the stillness will draw you in and you can try some of the other forms found in the section on meditation (page 150).

Try not to spend too much time on the addictions of the Internet and computer games, or even the addiction of work on your computer. Computers launch the mind into cyberspace, and if there is one thing that Vata does not need it is more space! Likewise, all intellectual activity provokes Vata. So if you are a student and your constitution is Vata, take care to have breaks at regular intervals for a different kind of activity that is more body-based.

In terms of making a living in the world, Vata is brilliant at spontaneously conjuring up creative ideas. This is all well and good, but having to come up with them to order and with the spectre of a deadline looming is Vatagenic! Also, often these creative wonders lack the fire to put their ideas into practice and the determination to follow through. For some Vata types working in a team with a good blend of Pitta and Kapha will provide the necessary drive and determination.

Lastly, enjoy a relaxing holiday. Do not book another Mongolian trek or a trip canoeing up the Zambesi. Go for sun, sea and sleep.

FOR THE PITTA TYPE

The Pitta person needs to be treated like one's spouse, say the seers. I would interpret that as treating Pitta as an equal partner with fairness and love. Do that with yourself; do not be judgemental. Neither you nor anyone else needs judging; it does not make us shine. Treat yourself and others with compassion.

Unlike Vata, usually you need to loosen up a bit with the scheduling and forget the timetable occasionally. That will be hard due to your innate desire to organize and control yourself and everything else. But, since your mind is extremely logical, you will find it easier if you understand the need to indulge your spontaneity every so often.

Make sure you are not too hot in bed and have opaque coverings at the open windows to admit air but occlude the light (particularly as the nights get shorter) because you sleep lightly and you are very sensitive to light.

Your main addiction is very likely 'work', so you too need relaxation. Oils that can cool and relax are found on pages 143–5. Some Pitta people do not like the feeling of too much oil on the skin, so lighter creams may be used in massage or reflexology. Oil feeds fire; it provides a barrier to evaporating moisture and heat, both of which are Pitta qualities.

You usually have excellent stamina and so if you are sufficiently tired to think of taking a daytime nap, take a good look

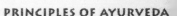

at your health. If you live somewhere hot or are on holiday you might need a nap in the cool shade after a large meal or when the sun is at its highest.

Mix with friends whose company you enjoy because they are stimulating but who do not provide hooks for your innate competitiveness – perhaps those whose expertise is in fields other than your own.

Pitta too needs periods away from the chalk face. Pitta needs to remember that leisure is for relaxation, not for learning another skill. Things that appeal to Pitta are often visually orientated like the creative arts, particularly painting. Try taking up one of these activities for the pure joy of creating, and watch for tell-tale signs of wanting to be the best! Gardening, with the addition of a challenge like specialist plant-growing or garden design, might appeal.

If you are not used to any form of meditation, again the best way is to timetable in five minutes or so daily to build a new habit. The early morning and evening Vata times are the best times for meditation, as the quality of 'subtle' promotes good meditation.

You do not have the problem of finding it difficult to organize yourself like the Vata person; your problem is accepting that work can be delayed, and indeed benefits from the time given to meditation. Meditation that is good for Pitta can be introduced using the sense that is most closely allied to that Dosha: sight. Sitting contemplating a candle flame or using a tape that talks you through a visualization (Pitta is usually adept at this form of internal sight) is a good way to begin. Other meditations can be found on page 150.

The Pitta digestion is good, as the fires of digestion burn brightly. However, it is necessary to eat regularly to avoid the hypoglycaemia (low blood sugar) that the unprepared Pitta person can experience in the form of irritability, nausea or wooziness. Carrying a small bag of fruit and nuts can keep you going if a meal is unavoidably delayed. Do not substitute chocolate bars or other sweet snacks for the fruit and nuts. Their refined sugars are absorbed rapidly, boost the blood sugar levels suddenly and cause insulin to be released from the pancreas to remove the excess sugar. This swinging about of sugar levels can be prevented by using unrefined sugars such as those found in fruits, etc., which break down and are absorbed into the bloodstream slowly, sustaining normal blood sugar levels. Diet is dealt with in a later section.

Exercise is another area that needs careful choosing to avoid provoking the Pitta trait of competitiveness. Pittas generally have good stamina and physiques, and need to feel somewhat challenged. So choose a form of exercise that is challenging (so you avoid boredom) but is not pitting you against another. Skiing on snow is excellent as it takes great skill and uses your developed musculature and coordination, and takes place in a cold location. Some other forms of exercise that would benefit a Pitta individual long term are kayaking, windsurfing and track and racket sports.

In the sphere of work and career Pitta people have a hard time not being successful – personally and financially. If they fail in their own eyes (even that phrase of judgement uses the Pitta-related sense of sight) they can become very depressed – and Pitta depression can be dangerous! It is also true that it is hard for them not to succeed, as they are ambitious, driven, efficient, incisive and decisive. Employment that makes good use of quintessentially Pitta qualities includes executive management, financial advising, the legal profession and medical, scientific and academic research.

When, eventually, you are forced to take a holiday (it is either that or divorce and ill-health) the type of break that suits you best is active and stimulating enough to engage your physical and mental energy but much less organized than your daily round. Go touring in Scandinavia, go trekking in Nepal, visit places of interest in your favourite country, but do not plan the route too much ahead – see what desires arise spontaneously each day. You might even get a taste for it if you spend a couple of days relaxing with a good book. Discuss annual holidays with Vata and Kapha friends and consider their ideal breaks with minor modifications.

FOR THE KAPHA TYPE

The Vedic seers advised treating the Kapha person 'like your enemy'. By advocating 'harsh' rather than 'soft' treatment they were addressing the Kapha type's need of motivation and stimulation. Generally, Kapha needs a bit of a push to get the rock rolling and a hefty nudge every now and again to change course, as the rolling rock may not be gathering moss but it does keep on in the same groove.

Sleep and Kapha are literally good bedfellows. Try getting a Kapha person up in the morning even with the prospect of a treat ahead. Try doing some necessary but not much desired exercise in the evening and your sleep will be well justified. Sleep under a light but warm duvet with the window ajar. Buy an insistent alarm clock or take a persistent partner who will not let you sleep right through the Kapha morning time (6–10 a.m.). If you lie in you will awake with a heavy head, be congested and sinusey, feel even less like starting the day and want to go back to sleep.

Relaxation must be just that for you, which means you must be sure that you are taking a break from something and not making it an entire lifestyle. You, of all the Doshic types, have the physical and mental constitution that would enable you to fully participate in the Vatagenic contemporary world culture and still have a nervous system that is not in tatters. But generally you don't want to. Unfair, isn't it?

The massage that suits you best is active and stimulating; deep tissue, therapeutic massage. If oils are used, check the aromatherapy section (page 143) for suitable ones. Essential oils may be used in the bath and bedroom to help with Kapha catarrhal, chest and sinus conditions and to give you a bit of pep in the mornings.

Unless you are physically ailing, *do not sleep* during the daytime. It will leave you feeling much the same as sleeping in too long, and you will find it really difficult to shake off the lethargy.

Kapha digestion is very efficient and slow. Your digestive system does extract everything possible from the food you eat – but slowly. The proverbial putting on weight just by looking at a cream cake applies to you. You do not need snacks between meals and should indeed remember that it takes three hours plus for the stomach to empty after a meal. More food should not be put in before the last lot has moved on. Eating lightly and using the spices listed in the section on diet will aid the digestion and help stop that heavy feeling after eating.

Your most likely addiction is to food, often as compensation for perceived lack of affection (look at the Dhatus and note that Meda/fat tissue gives us that feeling of being loved). Seek out company that supports and nurtures you as well as providing you with some stimulation. People who encourage you to be active are also to be wooed. You are not usually a talkative type, so doing an activity that you would enjoy with people you like and who share your enthusiasm is a good way to socialize. Combining this with something that uses your inborn physical strength and stamina, like long-distance walking or climbing, would be beneficial.

Because you are dependable and so good at smoothing ruffled feathers, team sports and activities like climbing allow you to exhibit wonderfully positive Kapha qualities and give you the motivation to continue. If you do not exercise at all at present, join the local ramblers group (one that does graded walks) and enjoy being out in the elements and letting the elements feed you. Your warm, compassionate, earthy disposition will soon ensure that other group members look forward to your company and remind you about prospective walks. You too can enjoy gardening, being at one with the earth. The more strenuous aspects of this activity will use up much of the stored energy that Vata people lack and would so love to have.

If Vata finds it impossible to create a routine (life is so full of surprises and one has to be ready to embrace them all) and Pitta organizes everything and everyone (only by controlling the world can things get done), Kapha has a routine that is the route to a rut! Try a tiny change in your usual timetable. Vary something small, just try it and see that the world will still turn on its axis and that you feel a little more alive. Phone your most Vata friend and arrange to spend a few hours together (could either of you cope with more?).

Meditation has a place in Kapha's life too, but make sure that you sit with your spine erect and that you choose a time when you are fully awake, to minimize the possibility of dropping off. Though early morning is generally the best time to meditate, before the activity of daily life builds up, it is probably best for you to use the early evening Vata time of 2 to 6 p.m. if you are just introducing meditation into your daily regime. Later you could try another session early in the day. Also, the use of incense will appeal to the Kapha person, as the sense of smell has such a strong affinity with Earth. The smell of incense will become a stimulus to which your mind and body become conditioned, and the peace and calm of meditation will be enhanced – more on this in the section on mantra and meditation (page 150).

In the realm of work Kapha brings consistency, diplomacy, perseverance, empathy and caring. The arenas best suited to making the most of Kapha's strengths are the caring professions like counselling and nursing, office management, construction work, conservation and archaeology, and the hotel and catering services.

When you take a holiday include some activities that stimulate you, body and mind. A walking holiday, sailing in a small craft convoy round the Greek islands or touring with some sightseeing done on foot are all good options; and you can always opt for an additional few days of self-indulgence on a beach or by a lake.

DIET: YOU ARE (TO A GREAT EXTENT) WHAT YOU EAT

Let me recap the information about the six tastes introduced in Chapter 3 before examining the foods that are best suited to each Dosha.

Sweet, sour and salty pacify Vata,
Sweet, bitter and astringent soothe Pitta.
Pungent, bitter and astringent soothe Kapha.
The therapeutic effects of tastes are as follows:

- Sweet is mildly cooling, the most moistening, and adds the most heaviness. It is nutritive, strengthening and balancing to the mind and soothing to the body's mucous membranes (the protective membranes that line organs such as the stomach, intestines, mouth and gullet). It calms down burning sensations.

- Sour is moderately heating, mildly moistening, and increases lightness to the greatest extent. It is stimulating to the palate and to saliva. It dispels flatulence, improves circulation (is heating) and is nutritive to tissues (with the exception of the reproductive tissues).

- Salty is mildly heating, moderately moistening, and is moderately heavy. It is stimulating to the digestive tract – in small amounts promoting digestion, in medium amounts acting as a cathartic and in large amounts causing vomiting. It is sedative to the nervous system.

- Pungent is the most heating and drying of tastes and has a moderately lightening effect. It has a generally stimulating effect on digestion, metabolism and circulation. Therefore it is useful in flatulence, colic, indigestion and poor circulation, and to induce sweating in fevers.

- Bitter is the most cooling and lightness-inducing, and is moderately drying. It reduces fevers, kills bacteria and parasites and, in small amounts, stimulates the secretion of digestive juices. To this end it is commonly an ingredient of pre-dinner drinks (as in Angastura bitters).

- Astringent is moderately cooling and moderately heaviness- and dryness-inducing. It has a contracting effect on tissues and thus stops bleeding, diarrhoea, catarrhal discharges, sweating and inflammation.

The six tastes are found mixed in substances but in differing amounts. The predominant tastes in some common foods are listed opposite.

TASTE	FOODS/FOOD CATEGORIES
Sweet	Sugars (cane and beet), fruit sugars (e.g. date sugar), milk sugar, maple syrup, molasses, honey. Also in fats and complex carbohydrates such as grains and root vegetables.
Sour	Acidic fruits such as the citrus fruits and tomatoes, and sour varieties of other fruits such as apples, berries, plums and grapes. All fermented foods such as pickles, vinegar and alcohol.
Salty	All sea food (including seaweeds) and sea and rock salts.
Pungent	Tea, coffee and spices such as ginger, cinnamon, black pepper, cayenne pepper and paprika.
Bitter	Though not a predominant taste in foods (indeed it is often a sign that a food is 'off'), it can be found in many medicinal herbs to good effect.
Astringent	Commonly predominant when fruits (such as bananas) are unripe. Predominant in pomegranates and lettuce.

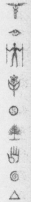

GENERAL ADVICE ON DIET AND DOSHA

If your scores for the Prakruti questionnaire indicate that you are a close mix of two Doshas or even a Tridoshic person, then you must take other information into account when making dietary choices. For example, a Vata/Pitta person should stick to the Vata diet during the seasons that are cold (remember, autumn is particularly Vatagenic) and should use Pitta-soothing foods in the summer and late spring. It is also important to take Vikruti (the state of imbalance) into account. Using diet to decrease the aggravated Dosha is a safe and effective if somewhat slower treatment than others that require more specialist knowledge.

It is because it is slow relative to herbal treatment, for example, that diet is so safe and radical (in the sense of getting to the root of a problem). Such effects are sure to be long lasting and give the mind as well as the body time to adjust. Generally, the body does not take well to drastic and speedily implemented changes. The body takes time to change its habits – foods and activities that it has become used to. A couple of consistent changes in how and what you eat are worth innumerable abortive attempts at changing your entire daily dietary regime.

Take care to remember that the food lists for each Dosha are given as general advice. You may be sensitive to certain foods and, of course, *must not eat them* just because you discover that your Doshic type *can* eat these foods. Also, foods that you are addicted to and that you would be miserable about dropping entirely can and should be reduced in quantity and frequency rather than eliminated entirely, at least initially. Removing items suddenly may provoke reactions, particularly if you start to reintroduce them after a period of withdrawal.

As an example, think of the case of a person who is sensitive to dairy but who may not actually be aware of this because he has always loved it and eaten it every day. The catarrhal congestion he has experienced for years has been an inconvenience he has grown to accept. Because he is predominantly Kapha he decides to eliminate dairy from his diet and does so consistently from the day he makes his decision. After a few days he may find that he craves the eradicated foods and that he is getting headaches as his body, released from the daily dose of dairy, turns the energy previously used to cope with a state of allergy to eliminate accumulated wastes. If he stays with it these symptoms may diminish and, after a few months, he may forget how bad he used to feel and decide to reintroduce his beloved dairy ('After all, where's the harm in it?'). Rather rapidly he may feel worse than he did before he tried cutting dairy out of his diet as his body rebounds in its reaction to a substance it is sensitive to. Be kind to yourself, this is not a punishment and feeling miserable is not conducive to health.

Be aware that it is your daily diet that counts – the occasional indiscretion is dealt with by a healthy person. Make up the bulk of your diet from fresh, seasonal, organically grown, non-genetically modified foods. Home-grown and home-cooked are best – think of the love that is being ingested along with the food. In Eastern traditions the position of cook is revered and honoured, as someone who is well progressed on the spiritual path has the most to add to the diets of those he cooks for.

Too much food is merely converted into Ama. What constitutes 'too much' is determined by the state of your digestion – therefore, if you are Vata or have a Vata imbalance, eat small meals and watch for signs of not digesting properly. Foods cooked together such as soups and stews are generally most easily digested.

Food combining is an important subject in Ayurveda. Here are some general combinations to avoid:

- Fruit is a food that is best eaten on its own. That is, you can mix fruits that are suitable for you, but do not have them at the same sitting as other types of food. It makes a good breakfast or you can have it as a mid-morning or mid-afternoon snack.
- Sour dairy such as yoghurt should not be eaten at the same meal as sweet dairy such as milk or cream.

- Raw foods such as salads or muesli should not be taken at the same meal as cooked foods.
- Dairy should not be eaten with starches.

Apart from drinking a little water or a small amount of wine with a meal, drinks are best taken between meals. The rule is one-third fluid, one-third food and one-third empty to allow good mixing.

Do not exercise until a couple of hours have elapsed after a meal, apart from a short stroll enabling the contracting and relaxing abdominal muscles to massage the intestinal contents as you walk. The process of digestion takes energy, the activity of a specific part of the nervous system and blood flow to the digestive organs, all of which necessitate a certain degree of passivity in other parts of the body and mind.

Finally, remember that food is intended to supply Prana in a gross form, to nourish the body and maintain its physical existence, while the subtle components of food feed the mind. As the subtle energies that enter the organism are so important, always eat mindfully. Eating while watching television, reading the paper or having a heated discussion will compromise digestion and permit these materials to be absorbed along with the food – bitter fruits indeed!

ANIMAL PRODUCTS

VATA

YES

AVOID

All are good in moderation
for grounding Vata. The dark
meat of chicken and turkey in
preference to the white meat.

PITTA

YES

Chicken (white meat)

Egg whites

Fresh water fish

Rabbit

Turkey (white meat)

Venison

AVOID

All other animal products
including egg yolks

KAPHA

YES

Chicken (white meat)

Eggs

Freshwater fish

Rabbit

Turkey (white meat)

Venison

AVOID

Beef

Duck

Lamb

Pork

Sea fish/food

CONDIMENTS

VATA

YES   AVOID

Most   Horse radish
Chocolate (occasionally)
Chilli peppers (in moderation)

PITTA

YES   AVOID
Black pepper (occasionally)   All others including:
Coriander leaves   Chillis
Mango chutney (sweet)   Chutneys
Lime, fresh (occasionally)   Horse radish
Salt (in moderation)   Mustard
                                       Lemon
                                       Mayonnaise
                                       Pickles
                                       Tomato
                                       Ketchup
                                       Vinegar

KAPHA

YES   AVOID
Black pepper   Chutneys (sweet)
Chilli pepper   Pickles
Coriander leaves   Mayonnaise
Horseradish   Salt
Ketchup (occasionally)   Soya sauce
Lemon (in moderation)   Tamari

Mango chutney (spicy)   Vinegar
Mustard
Seaweeds (in moderation)

CULINARY HERBS AND SPICES

VATA

YES   AVOID
All spices

PITTA

YES   AVOID
Black pepper (occasionally)   All others
Caraway (occasionally)
Coriander leaves
Cumin
Dill
Fennel
Ginger, fresh
Mint
Orange peel (occasionally)
Parsley (occasionally)
Peppermint
Saffron
Spearmint
Turmeric
Vanilla (occasionally)

YES

AVOID

All spices
Fennel (in moderation)
Vanilla (in moderation)

DAIRY FOOD

VATA

YES

AVOID

All fresh dairy.
Dilute and add spices to
yoghurt
Ice cream (in moderation)

All dried products and yoghurt
with fruit

PITTA

YES

AVOID

Light and sweet
Milk
Cottage cheese
Cream
Ghee

Salty and sour
Buttermilk
Hard cheese
Salted butter
Sour cream
Yoghurt

KAPHA

YES

AVOID

Ghee (in moderation)
Unsalted goats' cheese
Goat's milk (in moderation)

Most

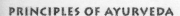

VATA

YES	AVOID
Juices:	
Apricot	Apple
Berry (except cranberry)	Mixed veg
Carrot	Pear
Cherry	Pomegranate
Grape	
Grapefruit	
Mango	
Orange	
Peach	
Pineapple	
Hot Drinks:	
Chai (hot, spiced milk)	Caffeinated tea/coffee
Grain coffee	Chocolate
Soya milk (hot, spiced)	Cocoa
Cold Drinks:	
Almond milk	Carbonated iced drinks
Fresh lemonade	Soya milk (cold)
Alcoholic Drinks:	
Beer (in moderation)	Spirits
Cider (in moderation)	
Wine (in moderation)	
Herb Teas:	
Most, the following occasionally:	
Jasmine	Blackberry
Lemon balm	Ginseng
Nettle	

Passion flower
Strawberry
Mate
Raspberry (in moderation)

PITTA

YES	AVOID
Juices:	
Apple	Carrot
Apricot	Cranberry
Grape	Grapefruit
Mango	Orange
Mixed veg	Pineapple
Peach	Sour berry
Pear	Sour cherry
Sweet berry	Tomato
Sweet cherry	
Hot Drinks:	
Bouillon	Caffeinated tea/coffee
Chai (occasionally, hot,	Chocolate
spiced)	Cocoa
Grain coffee	
Cold Drinks:	
Almond milk	Iced drinks
Carob milk	Lemonade
Cows' milk	
Lassi (diluted yoghurt)	
Rice milk	
Soya milk	
Alcoholic Drinks:	
Beer (occasionally)	Cider
	Spirits

Herb Teas:
Most

Cinnamon
Ginger (dried)
Ginseng
Hawthorn
Rosehip
Mate

KAPHA

YES   AVOID
Juices:
Apple   All sour
Apricot
Berry
Carrot
Cherry, sweet
Cranberry
Mango
Mixed veg
Peach
Pear
Pomegranate
Hot Drinks:
Caffeinated tea/coffee
  (in moderation)
Grain coffee
Soya milk (hot, spiced)
Veg bouillon
Cold Drinks:
Carob drinks   Rice milk
                       Soya milk (cold)
                       Iced drinks

Alcoholic Drinks:

Cider	Beer
Wines (dry)	Spirits
	Wines (sweet)

Herb Teas:
Most, the following
moderately:
Comfrey
Fennel
Ginseng
Liquorice
Rosehip (occasionally)

FRUIT

VATA

YES	AVOID
Most sweet fruit. If in doubt,	All dried
cook. If dried, soak overnight	Apples (raw)
and preferably cook.	Cranberries
	Pears
	Watermelon

PITTA

YES	AVOID
Most sweet and astringent	Sour fruit and sour varieties:
fruit, including dried.	Apricots
Also:	Berries
Grapes (except green)	Cherries
Limes (in moderation)	Oranges
	Pineapples
	Plums

YES
Most astringent and dried
fruit
Figs (dried, in moderation)
Grapes (in moderation)
Lemons (in moderation)
Limes (in moderation)
Mangos (occasionally)

AVOID
Most sour and sweet fruit,
including:
Coconut
Figs, fresh

GRAINS

VATA

YES
Cooked:
Durham wheat
Oats (cooked)
Quinoa (in moderation)
Rice (vary all types)
Rice cakes (occasionally)
Wheat pasta (occasionally)

AVOID
Dry as in muesli/breakfast
  cereals:
Barley
Buckwheat
Maize
Millet
Oats (dry)
Oat bran
Rye
Sago
Spelt
Tapioca
Wheatbran

YES	AVOID
Barley	Buckwheat
Oats (cooked)	Maize
Oat bran	Millet
Rice (brown, only	Oats (raw)
occasionally)	Quinoa
Sago	Rye
Spelt	
Tapioca	
Wheat	
Wheat bran (in moderation)	

KAPHA

YES	AVOID
Barley	Oats (cooked)
Buckwheat	Rice (brown/white)
Durham wheat	Wheat grains
Maize	Wheat flour
Millet	
Quinoa (in moderation)	
Rye	

NUTS AND SEEDS

VATA

YES   AVOID
All nuts and seeds
(in moderation)
Sesame seeds (roasted)

PITTA

YES   AVOID
Almonds (skinned,
occasionally)   All nuts
Pumpkin seeds (roasted,
in moderation)   Sesame seeds
Sunflower seeds (roasted,
in moderation)

KAPHA

YES   AVOID
Coconut   All nuts
Pumpkin seeds (roasted,
in moderation)
Poppy seeds
Sesame seeds
Sunflower seeds (roasted,
in moderation)

OILS/FATS

VATA

YES   AVOID

All oils except blended
vegetable oil

PITTA

YES	AVOID
Canola	Almond
Coconut	Animal fats
Olive	Corn
Sunflower	Sesame (dark)
Safflower (in moderation)	
Soya (in moderation)	
Walnut	

KAPHA

YES	AVOID
Small amounts only of:	Most, especially:
Canola	Apricot
Corn	Avocado
Ghee	Coconut
Safflower	Olive
Sunflower	Sesame
	Soya
	Walnut

PULSES

VATA

YES | AVOID
Mung dhal | Most, including soya flour and
Red lentils | cold tofu
Soya derived products:
Milk
Cheese
Sauce
Sausages
Tofu (cooked)

PITTA

YES | AVOID
Most, especially: | Fermented products such as
Aduki | Miso and soy sauce
Mung dhal
Tofu (cooked)
due to their Sattvic influence
on the mind.

KAPHA

YES | AVOID
Most pulses | Soya beans and their products
Soya milk (best spiced) | including cold tofu
Tofu (cooked only)

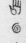

SWEETENERS

Honey must be used uncooked as heated it produces Ama.

VATA

YES   AVOID
Most   Saccharin
                        White sugar

PITTA

YES   AVOID
Most   In excess:
                        Jaggary
                        Honey
                        Molasses
                        Saccharin
                        White sugar

KAPHA

YES   AVOID
Honey (in small amounts) All others
is best. Also, but sparingly:
Barley malt
Brown rice syrup
Fruit juice concentrates
Maple syrup

VEGETABLES

VATA

YES	AVOID
Well cooked. Use spices and add ghee as a condiment.	Raw and cold as in salads.
Artichoke	Aubergine
Asparagus	Bell peppers
Black olives	Brussels sprouts
Broccoli (occasionally)	Celery
Cabbage (occasionally)	Green olives
Carrots	Kohlrabi
Cauliflower (occasionally)	Leeks (uncooked)
Courgettes	Lettuce
Daikon radish	Mushrooms
Fennel	Onion (raw)
Green beans	Potatoes (white)
Kale (occasionally, well cooked)	Turnips
Leeks (cooked)	
Onions (cooked)	
Pumpkin	
Parsnips (in moderation)	
Radishes	
Spinach (in moderation)	
Sprouts (in moderation)	
Squashes (in moderation)	
Sweet corn (in moderation)	
Sweet potato	
Tomatoes (occasionally)	

YES	AVOID
Most sweet and bitter veg	Pungent veg
Only cooked:	
Beets	Chillis
Carrots	Garlic
Leeks	Mustard greens
Onions	Tomatoes
Radishes	Turnips
Spinach (occasionally)	
Sweet corn (occasionally)	
Also, cooked or uncooked,	
as suitable:	
Artichoke	
Asparagus	
Broccoli	
Brussels sprouts	
Cabbage	
Cauliflower	
Cucumber	
Endive	
Green beans	
Kale	
Ladies fingers	
Lettuce	
Parsnips	
Peas	
Potatoes	
Sprouts	
Sweet peppers	
Squashes	
Watercress	

YES	AVOID
Most pungent and bitter veg	Sweet and watery veg
Artichoke	Courgettes
Aubergine	Cucumber
Asparagus	Mushrooms
Bean sprouts	Pumpkin
Cabbage	Squashes
Carrots	Sweet potatoes
Cauliflower	Tomatoes (raw)
Celery	Also, sour, pungent and salty
Daikon radish	veg such as olives and pickles
Fennel (in moderation)	
Garlic	
Green beans	
Kale	
Ladies fingers	
Leeks	
Mustard greens	
Onions	
Peas	
Spinach	
Turnips	
Watercress	

There are some very useful textbooks that can give you more detailed information and advice on diet, including suitable menus for the Doshic types. Several of these are listed in the Bibliography. Please investigate these and implement the cumulative suggestions, because consistent dietary changes alone will have a profound effect on your well-being – given that all-important element of time.

TAKE A BREAK – MAKE A FAST

If what you eat is important in Ayurveda, then so is what and when you *avoid* eating. Fasting has an honourable and venerated place in lifestyle and treatment as recommended by traditional Ayurveda. And, as with almost everything else, how you go about it depends upon your constitution.

If Vata is your Prakruti or is the Dosha that is vitiated, then the hot-house plant technique should be applied – easy does it! About once a fortnight choose a day when you can take it easy and avoid solid food. Drink diluted fruit juices (check the food lists), spiced milk or lassi, or hot water with lemon and honey. Avoid trying to drink water alone and do not extend the fast.

If Pitta is your type or is deranged, then take a day a week to eat a mono diet. This is when you rest the digestive tract by eating only one sort of foodstuff such as grapes, but you eat them in the quantity you desire. Pitta also benefits from eating raw fruit or raw vegetable salads only, or their diluted juices. A third type of fast that suits Pitta is eating kichadi only. This can be extended for several days but not beyond feeling that you never want to look a mung bean in the face again! As with Vata, do not indulge in water-only fasts.

Kapha digestion benefits greatly from regular weekly fasts taking only suitable juices or warm water and (the unfairness of it!) Kapha can undertake longer fasts, particularly at the turn of the seasons.

ADDITIONS TO YOUR SELF-HELP MANUAL

The Ayurvedic concept of 'medicine' includes anything and everything that will increase well-being by contributing to bringing the whole person into a dynamic balance. The emphasis on 'dynamic' rather than 'static' affirms the notion of change as fundamental to human existence. Thus the huge importance given to daily regimen and daily diet to help keep the ever-changing self on as even a keel as possible as it sails through life.

The journey, of course, includes stormy times that demand different foods and routines and even visits to health professionals for the kind of help we looked at in Chapter 7. Here are some things we can add to the diet/lifestyle foundation to enhance the beauty of being alive: household herbs, aromatherapy, colour and gem therapy, mantra and meditation, and yoga.

HOUSEHOLD HERBS

There are several culinary herbs and spices that you will probably have in a cupboard which can be used in self-help Ayurveda. Perhaps you already keep a few other substances, such as ghee, that will be useful in Ayurvedic cooking and can be used as household cures. Very likely the difference between how you

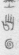

have hitherto used them and how you can use them for self-healing is to do with quantity and frequency.

BLACK PEPPER

Black pepper can be used to good effect as follows:

Black pepper will decrease Vata and Kapha but increase Pitta, so watch out for signs of high Pitta like redness, heat, irritability or anger.

- A pinch of black pepper with a teaspoonful of honey *acts as a natural antihistamine and is very good for sinus congestion.*
- In a mixture with ginger and long pepper (Trikatu or three peppers) *it increases Agni (digestive fire), improving appetite and digestion.*
- A pinch with a teaspoonful of ghee is *anti-allergy and therefore useful for symptoms of the hay fever variety.*

TURMERIC

Turmeric, the yellow root powder used in the preparation of curries, is a powerful antibiotic. It helps kill off viruses, bacteria, fungal organisms and even worms. It has many uses:

- *For chronic bronchitis:* 1 teaspoonful in a cup of milk, boiled and taken daily.
- *For a sore throat:* 1 teaspoonful in a cup of milk, boiled and taken daily.
- *For iron-deficiency anaemia:* ¼ teaspoonful in a cup of yoghurt.
- *For eczema, dermatitis or psoriasis:* Make a paste with ghee and apply. Cover with care to avoid yellowing your clothes and bedding!

- *For fungal infections of nails or athlete's foot:* 1 teaspoonful of Aloe vera gel and ¼ teaspoonful of turmeric. Apply and cover.

ASAFOETIDA

Asafoetida is also used to flavour curries. The smell and taste of it is sulphurous, so you may regard the cure as worse than the problem! – but it can be used in self-help:

- *For chronic dyspepsia (indigestion):* 1 teaspoonful of ghee with a pinch of asafoetida.
- *For sexual debility:* 1 teaspoonful of ghee with a pinch of asafoetida.
- *Cavities:* Until you can get dental treatment for a cavity, use a toothpick to fill the offending hole with asafoetida powder.

GINGER

Ginger is the digestive aid *par excellence*:

- *To sharpen appetite and aid digestion:* Chew a sliver of fresh ginger before meals.
- *To relieve trapped gas or colicky pains:* Make a tea with ⅛ – ¼ teaspoonful of ginger powder; sip. You can use 1 teaspoonful of grated fresh ginger and boil it for 5 minutes. Honey can be added before drinking ginger tea, but wait until it has cooled to drinking temperature.
- *For a fever that starts in the morning or evening with goosebumps and shaking, a generalized body ache, backache, constipation, stiff joints and a rapid pulse:* ⅓ teaspoonful ginger powder plus equal amounts of cumin powder and myrrh powder (which you probably will not have in your cupboard – yet!). Steep

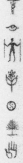

the herbs in a cup of hot water for 10 minutes before drinking. It will help induce a healing sweat to reduce the temperature.

- *For headache:* Make a paste with 1 teaspoonful of ginger powder and water, apply to the forehead and lie with it in place for half an hour. This can help some types of migraine too – try it.
- *For colds, cough, congestion, runny nose, post-nasal drip, fever with chills and dull heaviness in the head:* Take a tea of ginger, cinnamon and fennel. Make up a mixture of equal parts of these and store it in a tightly sealed jar in a cool, dark cupboard. When needed make a tea with 1 teaspoonful of the mixture in hot water, two to three times daily.

PIPPALI

If you can obtain pippali (long pepper) to use in trikatu (three peppers), then it can be used as follows:

- *For hayfever:* Make a tea with pippali, liquorice and lemongrass (powdered): ⅓ teaspoonful of each in hot water.
- *To help burn fat molecules:* Used alone or as trikatu, a pinch of the spice with 1 teaspoonful of honey, followed after 10 minutes by a cup of hot water and no other food or drink for at least one hour.
- *For Kapha conditions and problems where Ama is a major component, when you cannot obtain long pepper:* Make a mixture with 1 part bay leaves, ¼ part black pepper, ⅛ part cloves and 1/16 part cardamom. Use 1 teaspoonful to make 1 cup of the tea.

Using the list of herbs and spices given on pages 123–4, concoct mixtures that will benefit your Dosha or calm the Dosha

you know is increased. You can make your own tea bags of
herbs and spices – ground like ginger, whole like cloves and
cinnamon sticks, or as seeds like fennel or cumin – by making a
small bundle of the amount required in a square of unbleached
muslin. They are health- and environmentally-friendly and
recyclable.

AROMATHERAPY

Another beneficial addition to your balancing act is the use of
essential or volatile oils. A little was said about these wonderful
herbal extracts when we were looking at lifestyles, and suggestions were given as to how to use them (in oil burners, in baths,
on pads in your pillowcase at night, as steam inhalations or in
massage oil).

There are libraries full of books with good suggestions as to
how most effectively to combine these oils for various conditions of body and mind. Here I will restrict the advice given to
which oils are suited to each Dosha. In general, two to three
drops of two to three essential oils can be used in two treatments (say in a massage and in a bath) on the same day. *Never*
take volatile oils by mouth. Some practitioners are trained in
the internal use of essential oils and their advice can be followed, but for self-help purposes leave well alone. The reason
for this is the extremely concentrated nature of these oils.
Chemically they are oils but they do not appear oily. Their
intensity and oily nature are signatures of Pitta and they can
burn (only a very few essential oils can be used undiluted on
the skin, so do not use them except in a carrier oil, cream or
mixed well with bath water). Also, being so concentrated, very
little can be too much and taken internally can be very toxic.

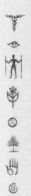

Oil	Dosha(s)
Camphor	Vata and Kapha
Cinnamon	Vata and Kapha
Eucalyptus	Vata and Kapha
Frankincense	Vata and Kapha
Lavender	Vata and Pitta
Lemon	Vata and Kapha
Lime	Pitta
Peppermint	Vata and Kapha
Rose, red	Vata
Rose, white	Pitta
Rose, yellow	Kapha
Rosemary	decreases Vata, Pitta (only if weak Agni), Kapha (for headaches)
Saffron	Vata, Pitta and Kapha
Sage	Vata and Kapha

Some other essential oils of particular benefit to each of the three Doshas include:

Vata	Cedarwood
	Geranium
	Juniper
	Myrrh
	Patchouli
	Ylang-ylang
Pitta	Gardenia
	Jasmine
	Lotus
	Sandalwood
	Vetivert
Kapha	Basil

Carrier oils for the Tridoshas differ, as they too have qualities that are needed by some types and best avoided by others.

Vata types can use oil of all varieties as the heaviness that is characteristic of all oils is grounding to Vata. However, good-quality cold-pressed sesame oil is warming to the Vata individual, and for this is particularly recommended by traditional Ayurveda. Castor oil is also very useful for Vata and is penetrating and healing. Light, gentle massage with long, flowing, stroking movements (effleurage) is beneficial to Vata.

Pitta needs far less oiling, but sunflower oil or coconut oil are recommended for their more cooling qualities when massage is required. More kneading and wringing movements can be incorporated into the massage for a Pitta individual, while keeping the stroking movements.

Kapha needs little oil, and indeed dry massage can be used to effect. If oil is used to facilitate the gliding of hands over skin, then use corn oil or mustard oil. Deep massage is good for Kapha using the friction of knuckles and thumb rotation as well as wringing and kneading movements.

The treatments dealt with so far have had their primary focus on the body – they are physical treatments. Those that follow are more subtle contributions to the restoration and mainte-nance of health. Treatments that are directed at the subtle bod-ies affect the physical body, as the subtle does not merely surround the body but suffuses it – anything that exists in the physical world must first exist in the subtle realms. Therefore, treatments that are directly connected to the subtle may work indirectly on the physical. Also, it may take time for the effects of these treatments to appear on the physical plane, and the cause-and-effect relationship may be more difficult to explain in what is termed 'scientific language'.

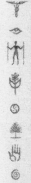

The philosophy (logical positivism) that lies behind Western science in the way that Sankhya philosophy underpins Ayurveda, ensures that only phenomena that can be subjected to experimental observation are deemed worthy of consideration. This has led to the acceptance of the ideal of the double-blind trial as the arbiter of scientific truth. Each of us has to decide for ourselves whether or not to accept the premises of this science as the only truth. Ayurveda (among several indigenous philosophies and sciences) offers other truths that do not force us to reject the Western scientific approach but invite us to see it as one among various important bodies of theory, each of which is useful in explaining some of the world around us.

COLOUR AND GEM THERAPY

The seven hues of the rainbow are cosmic colours which are connected with the Tridoshas through their constituent elements and their associated senses. Colour can be used to feed the mind and emotions through the sensations we absorb – and these, of course, affect the bodily Doshas.

These colours, used for their therapeutic value, can be brought into your life through the clothes you wear, the walls of the rooms you spend time in or, more specifically, by coloured light bulbs or filters such as paper stretched over windows, colouring all the incoming light. Similarly, water can be charged with the vibrations of particular colours by standing it in coloured glass vessels (or glass covered in coloured paper) in sunlight for several hours.

Vata is most positively affected by the colours red, orange and yellow, white and lighter shades of blue and green. Care should be taken with the frequency of use of red particularly, but also with any very strong, intense shades, because Vata is

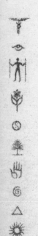

delicate. Paler shades are definitely recommended. Darker colours including grey, black and brown are to be avoided.

Pitta is benefited by the use of white, blue, green and purple, though again, avoid too strong or overly intense shades of these colours. Likewise, red and black are not recommended, though grey and brown are all right.

Kapha can take bright, stronger colours, especially the warmer tones of red, orange and yellow. Green, purple, brown, grey and black are acceptable, but dark blue can lead to congestion. Also, avoid white and the pastel shades of blue, pink and green.

The more natural the source of colour, the more replenishing, balancing and strengthening the effect. Therefore, colour combined with the natural qualities of minerals imbued with that colour (gemstones) is going to be extremely potent. The effect of gemstones will often be similar to that of other sources of colour, but some stones have a *Prabhava*, which means that the expected effect of their colour will be over-ridden by the special effect of their individual nature.

Gemstones may be used in rings and necklaces, or steeped in a glass of water overnight, then removed next morning so the water can be drunk. Care must be taken to ensure that the stones are intact when they are to be worn, but pieces of gemstones can be used to make gem waters. If worn as jewellery, stones are most beneficial if set so that they touch the skin. Some of the more common gemstones are listed below, and the Doshas they beneficially affect indicated.

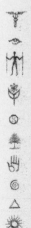

- Amethyst – contains the elements Ether and Water. Aids in balancing the emotions and in protecting healers (in the widest sense). It increases clarity of perception and spirituality. It has associations with the endocrine system. Wear it in gold around the neck. Benefits Vata and Pitta.

148

- Beryl – contains the elements Fire and Ether. Increases power and social position. It is associated with the visual arts and music. Wear it in silver as a ring on the left ring finger or around the neck. Benefits Vata and Kapha.
- Coral (Red) – contains the elements Fire, Water and Earth. It is balancing to Pitta despite its colour, and soothes Pitta emotions. It has a slightly Kaphagenic effect as it increases body muscle and it improves stamina. Good for Pitta and Vata but best avoided by Kapha.
- Diamond – contains all five elements. The gem water is a heart tonic and is rejuvenating. Also good in pregnancy. The stone is spiritually uplifting, increases creativity and creates close bonds in relationships as well as bringing prosperity. Wear it set in white gold or white and yellow gold mixed on the right ring finger. Diamonds particularly benefit Pitta (specifically the blue and white gems) but all diamonds can be used for Vata, though they may slightly increase Kapha.
- Emerald – contains Ether, Air and Water. It balances the nervous system, thereby affecting the mind (improving mental functioning) and the body (relieving pain). It is good for strengthening the pulmonary system, coronary circulation and the immune system. It restores balance and so is good for degenerative conditions. Wear it on the middle or little finger in silver for Pitta, or gold for Vata and Kapha (which it may slightly increase).
- Garnet – contains the elements Fire and Earth (red, brown and yellow garnets) or Fire and Air (green) or Water (white). Red, brown and yellow stones warm Vata and Kapha (set in gold and worn around the neck), while green and white stones set in silver reduce the heat of Pitta.
- Lapis lazuli – contains the elements Ether, Fire and Water. It has a strengthening effect on the body (particularly the eyes)

and mind, and increases spiritual awareness. Wear it in gold
around the neck. Good for Vata and Kapha.

- Moonstone – contains the elements Ether, Air and Water. As
  with the moon herself, the moonstone is closely associated
  with water in the body and with the emotions. It benefits
  those who are suffering from the effects of stress. Wear it set
  in silver on the right ring finger. Best for Vata and Pitta.
- Pearl – contains the elements Air, Water and Earth. Useful
  for all Pitta afflictions as it is cooling and promotes the
  Rakta/blood qualities of vitality and vigour. As a gem
  water made overnight it can be used to treat inflammatory
  conditions and acidity. Pitta should wear it set in silver on
  the right ring finger.
- Ruby – contains the elements Ether, Air and Fire. Ruby is
  good for the circulation and heart. It stimulates positive
  Pitta characteristics like good digestion and mental
  functioning. It brings decisiveness and confidence. Good for
  Vata and Kapha for its heating effect. Wear it set in either
  gold or silver (depending on the degree of warming
  required) on the ring finger of the left hand.
- Sapphire (Blue) – contains the elements Ether and Air. This
  stone has a particular association with Saturn (the god and
  the planet). It has an affinity with the nervous system and,
  though it is a dark blue colour to the naked eye, is useful in
  the Vata conditions – from neuralgia, nervousness and
  anxiety to ME and MS. It decreases Kapha-type problems
  like fatty deposits and over-attachment. Set it in silver or
  platinum and wear it on the middle finger or round the
  neck.
- Sapphire (Yellow) – contains the elements Ether, Fire and
  Water. Good to promote all-round health and vitality.
  Increases the production of Ojas. Increases spirituality and
  God consciousness. Can be used by all Doshas but is of

particular benefit to vitiated Vata as it increases centredness.
Wear it set in gold on the index finger.

MANTRA AND MEDITATION

'Man shall not live by bread alone...' Food feeds the physical
body, what we take in via the senses feeds the mind, and meditation feeds the spirit. Meditation should be an important part
of your daily routine – a part that feeds the spirit and which has
a knock-on beneficial effect on the mind and body. Listening to
the sound of silence is essential to wholistic living and is vital
to a lifestyle that supports the trinity of humanness – body,
mind, and spirit.

Food and the senses bring sustenance from the external environment, whereas in meditation your focus is internal. Since
you are in truth spirit in physical clothing and part of the One,
it is vital to your complete health to contact that One within by
regularly turning your focus inwards.

To meditate is to detach your awareness from external concerns and allow it to seek the God within. To facilitate this you
can use many tools, from focusing your attention on a candle
flame to the use of *mantra* (a Sanskrit word referring to sylla-
bles/sounds that have subtle energies). The point is to use
these tools in meditation to assist in easing the mind from its
usual treadmill of thoughts; therefore a main characteristic of
such tools is simplicity. Something that has many associations
will lead the mind off on another excursion. Therefore, visualization techniques and shamanic journeying, useful though
they are for contacting subtle parts of the Self, is not meditation. Talk to God by all means, regularly. Ask for blessings and
grace – this is supplicatory prayer. Ask also for blessings for
others – this is intercessionary prayer (and there are plenty of

examples of its beneficial effects). Use prayers of praise to express your gratitude for personal and global blessings. However, another aspect of communion with Spirit is allowing space and stillness of mind to receive the Divine response – this is meditation.

The usefulness of mantra in meditation is that the Sanskrit sounds produce subtle energies that reverberate with certain parts of our subtle bodies.

A simple mantra meditation is 'So-Hum'. In this meditation the 'So' syllable repeated internally on the in-breath represents universal consciousness, and the 'Hum' on the out-breath stands for 'self' consciousness. So-Hum is breathing in the universal and breathing out the ego. This is a meditation that can be used by anyone.

Sit comfortably, spine erect, on a cushion in the lotus or half-lotus posture or on a straight-backed chair, feet flat on the floor with the hands resting lightly on the thighs. Please be comfortable. If you cannot sit cross-legged without being painfully aware of it – don't!

Feel, imagine, visualize, 'intend' the breath rising from the base of the spine and moving up the front of the body through each *chakra* (Sanskrit for 'wheel' – see page 152). On reaching the crown chakra, pause and then breathe out while imagining the breath moving down through the third eye and crossing to descend the spinal column back to the base. The diagram overleaf shows how very easy this is.

Our problems as humans begin, as described in the Sankhya philosophy, with the belief in the myth of separateness. Our quest is to seek our own godliness within and thereby to unite and end the pain (physical, mental-emotional and spiritual).

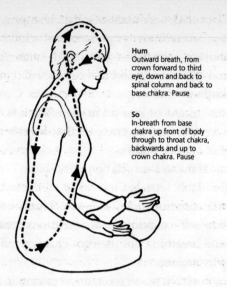

Hum
Outward breath, from crown forward to third eye, down and back to spinal column and back to base chakra. Pause

So
In-breath from base chakra up front of body through to throat chakra, backwards and up to crown chakra. Pause

So-Hum meditation

CHAKRAS AND MANTRAS

The Bija mantras (literally, seed mantras) are the sounds of the letters of the Sanskrit alphabet that are associated with the seven main chakras (energy centres of our subtle bodies that, of course, permeate and affect our physical existence). Because they permeate from the subtle to the gross of our existence, the chakras affect our physiology and our emotions. Below is a list of the seven main chakras in the order in which they exist, from the bottom of the spinal column to the crown of the head. They are envisaged as lotus flowers with varying numbers of petals. The main physiological and emotional associations of the various chakras and the primary Bija mantra relating to each is given. Benefit to the body and mind can be achieved by use of these simple mantras.

1   Root chakra (*Muladhara*), Earth element. It is centred at
    the base of the spine. Associated with the rectum,
    prostate, cervix and gonads. The main function of this
    energy centre is physical survival and groundedness.
    Ungroundedness is its dysfunction. Can lead to
    problems like food addiction (dissatisfaction associated
    with physical matter/Earth) and dysmenorrhoea. The
    Bija mantra is *Lam* and the associated colour and gem
    are red and the ruby respectively.

2   Self-Place (*Svadhisthana*), Water element. It is centred
    round the lower belly. Associated with the kidneys and
    adrenal glands. The main function of this centre is
    self-esteem, creativity (including reproduction) and
    personal sexuality. Its dysfunction manifests as
    over-attachment and low self-esteem. Can involve
    problems to do with fertility and premature ejaculation.
    The Bija mantra is *Vam* and the associated colour and
    gem are orange and red coral.

3   City of Gems (*Manipura*), Fire element. It is centred in
    the solar plexus and is associated with the digestive
    system including the pancreas. It has to do with the
    marriage of the male and female energies. Its functions
    are to do with personal power, dominating energy and
    competitiveness, and include the qualities of pride,
    confidence and achievement. The stress related to
    unfulfilled ambitions/lack of achievement can produce
    anger and hate as extremes of dysfunction. The Bija
    mantra is *LAM* and the colour and gem are yellow and
    the topaz.

4   The Heart Chakra (*Anahata*), Air element. Associated
    with the cardio-vascular system and the thymus gland
    (related to immunity). It is the bridge between the lower
    three bodily and 'tribal'-related chakras and the upper

three transpersonal ones. The main function is personal love of a higher nature than sex and it is the seat of love as an emotion and compassion. Its dysfunction is lack of love. Stress based here may be to do with rejected love. The Bija mantra is *YAM*, which is also the name of the god of death, in this instance the death of the Ego as the energy of Anahata bridges the lower Self and the higher Self. The colour is green and the gem is emerald.

5   Throat Chakra (*Vishuddha*), Ether element. This chakra is associated with the respiratory system and metabolism, and thus involves the thyroid and parathyroid glands. Its main functions are the expression of emotion and will-power, but all forms of communication are connected to this chakra, with the associated qualities of clarity and sharing. Unprocessed emotion can cause problems in this area, and lack of communication is its dysfunction. The Bija mantra is *HAM*, the colour is blue and the gemstone is the blue sapphire.

6   The Third Eye (*Agya* or *Ajna*), Consciousness is the element. It is centred behind the eyebrows and is associated with the ANS (Autonomic Nervous System, dealing with processes such as digestion which are usually beyond voluntary control) and the pituitary gland (the conductor of our hormonal system, which is the carrier of longer-lasting instructions to our body and emotions than the fast-acting nervous system). This is where gross and subtle, matter and mind meet and merge. The function is intuition and the dysfunction is refusal to see things as they really are. It works closely with the seventh chakra to keep logic and intuition balanced. The mantra is *SAM* (on the in-breath) and *KSHAM* (on the out-breath), the colour is indigo and the stone amethyst.

7 Crown Chakra (*Sahasrara*), Bliss is the element. It is centred on the pineal gland and holds sway over the CNS (Central Nervous System – activity of the brain and spinal cord). The seventh chakra's function is to initiate and stimulate the spiritual journey, to instil divine discontent so that we seek to transcend our physical human existence. Its dysfunction is mental imbalance, psychosis and depression. As stated in the previous paragraph, these two uppermost chakras of the body are where the logic of the left brain and the creativity and intuition of the right brain must balance and work together. Cold logic needs the warmth of love and compassion. We need the left brain's capacity for clear, abstract and logical thought but only in the service of spirit. The Bija mantra is *OM*, the colour violet and the stone the alexandrine.

You can work with the Bija mantras to help with the dysfunctions mentioned under each chakra. Envisage and feel the electro-magnetic current vibrating between the front and back of your body at each of the levels indicated by the descriptions of where the chakras are centred.

YOGA: BREATHING, EXERCISES AND THE DOSHAS

Yoga (meaning 'union') is another of the main Vedic sciences and as such has an age-old connection with Ayurveda. It is so much more than the exercise form that many of us in the West enjoy. Yoga is the ultimate in experiencing reality, as one of its main precepts states that only in uniting with whatever it is that you are trying to comprehend can you know it. As stated earlier, all human problems stem from not knowing our true

nature, which is as part of the great One. Thus Yoga and Ayurveda place knowledge of the true nature of Self and Reality at the centre of what it means to be healthy. Knowing oneSelf is essential to health. I encourage you to explore the science of Yoga, for here I only make certain health-giving and helpful suggestions.

In Ayurveda, Yoga *Asanas* (physical postures) and *Pranayama* (breath control) are often used therapeutically. These are only two of the eight branches of classical Yoga, but are the ones most directly affecting the physical body.

Asanas can be used to balance the Doshas generally or chosen for specific problems. Both Asanas and Pranayama (which works with the breath of life, Prana) boost vitality.

Vata individuals could benefit from alternate nostril breathing. Using the thumb and middle finger to open and close the two nostrils, first block one and breathe in through the other, then change over and breathe out. The next in-breath is via the same nostril you just breathed out through, and so it goes on.

Pitta people can reduce the heat and intensity of Pitta by breathing in via the left nostril and out via the right and repeating that sequence. Since the left nostril is related to the cool, compassionate, female, lunar energy it will induce related qualities in the individual.

Conversely, Kapha individuals who need the addition of some solar, masculine, heating, assertive energy should close the left nostril and breathe in through the right, release and breathe out via the left and continue that cycle.

Likewise, solar or lunar energy can be encouraged in the individual during sleep by lying on the left side (which blocks lunar energy) if Vata or Kapha are predominant, or choosing the right side (blocking solar energy) if Pitta is predominant. Similarly, lying on the right side will help reduce fever (should that be excessive) until more curative treatments can be given or taken.

Below are Yoga Asanas which are particularly suitable for problems related to each of the three Doshas. These are listed according to degree of difficulty. Postures that are useful for balancing each Dosha are in **boldface**. If you have never practised Yoga, find a good class locally (the Useful Addresses and Resources chapter will be of help) and learn the basics. You will probably find that the majority of postures mentioned will be incorporated in most Yoga classes. If you are in any doubt about a posture, ask for help and a demonstration.

VATA	PITTA	KAPHA
BASIC:	BASIC:	BASIC:
Cobra – helps with insomnia, constipation, spinal circulation and menstrual problems.	Boat – helps relieve gastritis, peptic ulcer and irritable bowel.	**Boat** – helps relieve sinus congestion and asthma. Useful in diabetes.
Corpse – conserves energy and balances blood pressure. Helps Vata type asthma, insomnia, depression and varicose veins.	**Bow** – stimulates the kidneys and neighbouring organs and the adrenals.	Bow – stimulates the kidneys and surrounding organs including adrenals. Helps in sinus congestion and asthma.
Forward Bend – improves circulation, particularly pelvic.	Bridge – relieves flatulence and constipation and stimulates spinal circulation.	Cobra – stimulates the kidneys and surrounding organs including the adrenal glands. It helps with constipation and asthma.
Knee to Chest – helps constipation and flatulence. Helps backache, sciatica.	Cobra – stimulates the kidneys and surrounding organs and the adrenal glands. Benefits high blood pressure.	Fish – improves asthma and other respiratory problems like bronchitis, sinus congestion with related headache and asthma.
Palm Tree – improves circulation, depression.	**Fish** – improves asthma, migraine, malabsorption and liver and respiratory problems.	
Pose of the Child – relieves constipation and improves circulation.	Knee to Chest – relieves flatulence and constipation.	

Yoga Mudra – tones nerve centres in the pelvis helping with menstrual problems. Alleviates headache and sciatica. Helps in depression.

INTERMEDIATE:

Locust – helps constipation and stimulates kidney function.

Plough – stimulates the thyroid and circulation and relieves constipation. Good for backache, headache, sciatica, menstrual disorders and depression.

Shoulder Stand – improves circulation, particularly in the upper body, and relieves constipation.

ADVANCED:

Head Stand – balances the nervous system. Helps varicose veins.

Lotus – tones pelvic nerve centres and helps in depression.

Locust – stimulates the kidneys and surrounding organs and the adrenals. The effects are increased if practised consecutively with the Bow and the Cobra. Also good for malabsorption.

Sheetali – encourages the flow of Prana and is cooling. Useful for peptic ulcer and migraine headaches.

INTERMEDIATE:

Shoulder Stand – improves thyroid function in hyperthyroidism. Benefits high blood pressure and migraines. Benefits the liver. Cools the emotion of anger.

ADVANCED:

Hidden Lotus – tones pelvic nerve centres. Helps with peptic ulcer and liver malfunction.

Forward Bend – tones the nervous system and facial muscles. Useful in bronchitis and diabetes.

Lion – rejuvenating, energizing and encourages the flow of Prana. Stimulating to the throat and larynx.

Palm Tree – improves circulation generally, warming. Good for asthma.

INTERMEDIATE:

Backward Bend – improves mobility, circulation and works on the nervous system. Helps with bronchitis and diabetes.

Plough – stimulates the thyroid. Relieves constipation and helps with sinus congestion and bronchtis.

Shoulder Stand – helps with asthma, emphysema and relieves constipation.

THE QUEST: HOW TO
FIND A THERAPIST AND
AND WHAT TO EXPECT

t should be clear by now that you can use Ayurveda to
design for yourself a lifestyle that will help re-create physically healthful harmony, maintain emotional balance and
provide guidance on a spiritual journey unaffiliated with any
organized religion. It has also been my intention to convey the
idea that there are times when the help of a professional should
be sought.

FINDING A QUALIFIED THERAPIST

In seeking a properly qualified therapist, keep the following in
mind. In the West to date the only people who are fully trained
Ayurvedic doctors (general practitioners of Ayurveda) are people from India or Sri Lanka who have completed a five-and-a-
half-year degree in Ayurvedic Medicine and Surgery, including
a period of internship at a teaching hospital. Those people will
have the letters F.A.M.S./B.A.M.S./D.A.M.S. after their names,
denoting Fellow/Bachelor/of Ayurvedic Medicine and Surgery,
or a Diploma in the same (indicating study in Sri Lanka).

There are various ways other practitioners can legitimately
include Ayurveda in their practice. As any 'new' therapy, philosophy or spiritual path is introduced into another culture

there will always be people who want to learn about it or train in it. People trained in alternative therapies or Western medicine are already seeking training in Ayurvedic science and skills. This training can be at several different levels but none of them is equivalent to being a qualified Ayurvedic physician, yet!

There are opportunities in other countries, for example South Africa, which has included Ayurveda in its legally specified medical choices (since 1994) and which provides courses for people who want to train as Pancha Karma technicians or Ayurvedic primary healthcare advisors. At the end of this text I have included some useful addresses, but the rate of growth of interest is so great that courses will be sprouting with increasing frequency throughout the West. Not all of these will be of an equally (or even sufficiently) high standard. These things are bound to happen before national or international regulation of a particular profession occurs.

Contact any umbrella organization for the alternative medical professions. Names and addresses of these are often found in healthcare periodicals available from your newsagent or local library. One of the best solutions is to canvass the opinion of anyone you know who has already sampled the wares. 'Word of mouth' is still among the most reliable guides. Also, check the qualifications of the named practitioner. Remember, Ayurvedic physicians have the letters mentioned above after their names. The professional status of other practitioners must be judged by whatever their primary qualification is. Therefore, look for qualifications in Western medical science, nursing, physiotherapy or pharmacy and also the main alternative therapies. The alternative medical professions such as homoeopathy, chiropractic, medical herbalism and osteopathy are fertile ground in which to seek people who are expanding their skills to include Ayurveda. Post-graduate training of such people (first for a certificate, then a diploma) will produce the first flowerings in the West of practitioners using Ayurveda.

Chapter 7 (and Chapters 8 and 9, to some extent) dealt with most of the therapies that an Ayurvedic practitioner would offer.

THE INITIAL CONSULTATION

A thorough initial consultation will include visual assessment of your gait, posture, skin and voice. An Ayurvedic physician should take your pulses and may look at your tongue, irises or urine. You will be questioned about your medical history and present state of health, including your appetite, digestion and bowel movements, as these are crucial indicators of the strength of Agni, the balance of the Tridoshas and the presence of Ama.

The practitioner may use your palm or your Jyotish chart (Vedic astrology) to help determine what is going on for you and the usefulness or otherwise of prescribing certain treatments at that particular time. In Ayurveda it is important to determine the right time as well as the right treatment; sometimes the best option is to do nothing (temporarily).

If it is deemed appropriate, herbs, diet, lifestyle (including exercise), Pancha Karma, meditation, oils, gems or colours (any or all) may be prescribed. Bon voyage!

BIBLIOGRAPHY

JYOTISH

DeFouw, Hart and Robert Svoboda, *Light on Life: An Introduction to the Astrology of India* (London: Arkana, 1996)

DIAGNOSIS AND THERAPIES IN AYURVEDA

Bhattacharya, A K, *Gem Therapy* (Calcutta: Firma KLM Private Ltd, 1985)

Johari, Harish, *Ayurvedic Massage: Traditional Indian Techniques for Balancing Body and Mind* (Rochester, VT: Healing Arts Press, 1996)

Joshi, Sunil V, *Ayurveda and Panchakarma: The Science of Healing and Rejuvenation* (Twin Lakes, WI: Lotus Press, 1996)

Lad, Vasant, *The Complete Book of Ayurvedic Home Remedies* (London: Piatkus, 1998)

—, *Secrets of the Pulse: The Ancient Art of Ayurvedic Pulse Diagnosis* (Albuquerque, NM: The Ayurvedic Press, 1996)

Mehta, Silva, Mehta, Mira and Shyam Mehta, *Yoga the Iyengar Way* (London: Dorling Kindersley, 1990)

Rendel, Peter, *Understanding the Chakras* (Wellingborough: Aquarian Press, 1990)

Ros, Frank, *The Lost Secrets of Ayurvedic Acupuncture* (Twin Lakes, WI: Lotus Press, 1994)

Sills, Franklyn, *The Polarity Process: Energy as a Healing Art* (Shaftsbury, Dorset: Element Books Ltd, 1989)

VanHowten, Donald, *Ayurveda and Life Impressions Body Work: Seeking Our Healing Memories* (Twin Lakes, WI: Lotus Press, 1996)

GENERAL AYURVEDA

Chopra, Deepak, *Ageless Body, Timeless Mind: A Practical Alternative to Growing Old* (London: Rider, 1993)

—, *Perfect Health: The Complete Mind/Body Guide* (London: Bantam Books, 1990)

—, *Quantum Healing: Exploring the Frontiers of Mind/Body Medicine* (New York: Bantam Books, 1989)

—, *Unconditional Life: Mastering the Forces that Shape Personal Reality* (New York: Bantam Books, 1991)

Frawley, David, *Ayurvedic Healing: A Comprehensive Guide* (Salt Lake City, UT: Passage Press, 1989)

—, *The Yoga of Herbs: An Ayurvedic Guide to Herbal Medicine* (Santa Fe, NM: Lotus Press, 1986)

Hope-Murray, Angela and Tony Pickup, *Healing with Ayurveda* (Dublin: Gill and Macmillan, 1997)

Lad, Vasant, *The Science of Self-Healing* (Santa Fe, NM: Lotus Press, 1985)

Morrison, Judith H, *The Book of Ayurveda* (London: Gaia Books Ltd, 1994)

Ranade, Subhash, *Natural Healing through Ayurveda* (Salt Lake City, UT: Passage Press, 1993)

Svoboda, Dr Robert E, *Ayurveda for Women: A Guide to Vitality and Health* (Newton Abbot: David & Charles, 1999)

—, *Ayurveda: Life, Health and Longevity* (London: Arkana, 1992)

—, *Prakruti: Your Ayurvedic Constitution* (Albuquerque, NM: Geocom, 1989)

Verman, Vinod, *Ayurveda: A Way of Life* (York Beach: Samuel Weiser, Inc., 1995)

TRADITIONAL TEXTS

Murthy, K R Srikantha (trans.), *Astanga Hrdayam* (vol. 1; Varanasi, India: Krishnadas Academy, 1991)

Sharma, R K and Bhagwan Dash, *Caraka Samhita* (vols I—III; Varanasi, India: Chowkhamba Sanskrit Series Office, 1992)

TANTRA

Svoboda, Robert E, *Aghora: At the Left Hand of God* (Albuquerque, NM: Brotherhood of Life, Inc., 1986)

—, *Aghora II: Kundalini* (Albuquerque, NM: Brotherhood of Life, Inc., 1993)

AYURVEDIC COOKING AND NUTRITION

Lad, Usha and Vasant Lad, *Ayurvedic Cooking for Self-Healing* (Albuquerque, NM: The Ayurvedic Press, 1994)

Morningstar, Amadea and Urmila Desai, *The Ayurvedic Cookbook: A Personalized Guide to Good Nutrition and Health* (Wilmot, WI: Lotus Light, 1991)

Tiwari, Maya, *Ayurveda, A Life of Balance: The Complete Guide to Ayurvedic Nutrition & Body Types with Recipes* (Rochester, VT: Healing Arts Press, 1995)

USEFUL ADDRESSES AND RESOURCES

UK

AYURVEDIC MEDICAL ASSOCIATION UK

General Secretary
Dr N S Sathiyamoorthty, D.A.M.S., D.Ac, PhD
59 Dulverton Road
Selsdon
Croydon CR2 8PJ
Tel: 020 8682 3876
Fax: 020 8333 7904
email: ayurvedic.asso@england.com
Maintains a register of qualified practitioners of Ayurveda and also of Siddha and Unani medicine.

The College of Ayurveda (UK) is the associated body recently established to run part-time post-graduate training (certificate and diploma) in Ayurveda. Involves weekend seminars over two years in London and six months at an Ayurvedic training establishment in India.

Contact:
Dr Mauroof Athique
Director of Studies
20 Annes Grove
Great Linford
Milton Keynes MK14 5DR
Tel: 01908 664518

THE AYURVEDIC TRADING CO. LTD

East-West Centre
10 High Street
Glastonbury BA6 9DU
Tel: 01458 833382
Fax: 01458 834236
email: greenway@globalnet.co.uk
website: www.eastwestcentre.com
Provides Ayurvedic herbs, formulas, prescriptions by mail order. Also books on Yoga, Ayurveda and Jyotish, and tapes of the American Sanskrit Institute. Workshops in Jyotish, Viniyoga, Ayurvedic massage, Indian head massage and Keralipyat (traditional martial art of South India).

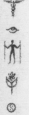

EAST WEST COLLEGE OF HERBALISM

Harts Wood
Marsh Green
Hatfield
East Sussex TN7 4ET
Tel: 01342 822312
Correspondence courses in Ayurveda and Vedic studies by Dr David Frawley.

THE HIMALAYA DRUG CO.
6 Chiltern Street
London W1M 1PA
Tel: 020 7935 0028
Supplier of Ayurvedic products from India to over 30 countries.

THE HIMALAYAN INSTITUTE
Peter Glover
70 Claremont Road
London W13 0DG
Tel/Fax: 020 8991 8090
Runs workshops and produces a Yoga magazine.

MAHARISHI AYUR-VED
Beacon House
Willow Walk
Skelmersdale
Lancashire WN8 6UR
Tel: 07000 AYURVEDA (298783)
Fax: 01695 50917
email: map@maharishi.co.uk
website: www.maharishi.co.uk
Offers consultations with Maharishi-trained practitioners. Also, foods, teas, oils and Maharishi Ayur-Ved products.

PRACTICAL AYURVEDA
Dr Ann Roden
27 Lankers Drive
North Harrow
Middlesex HA2 7PA
Tel: 020 8866 5944
Practical Ayurveda is a non-profit-making organization that runs one-day and weekend courses on the basic principles and practices of Ayurveda.

THE SIVANANDA YOGA CENTRE

51 Felsham Road
London SW15 1AZ
Tel: 020 8780 0160
Fax: 020 8780 0128
email: siva@dial.pipex.com
Teaches meditation and Yoga. Runs retreats and workshops on Ayurveda, Yoga and Sanskrit. Bookshop stocks books comprehensively covering these topics.

VINIYOGA BRITAIN

PO Box 158
Bath BA1 2YG
Tel/Fax: 01225 426327
Runs Yoga workshops, retreats and training courses.

THE WESSEX CENTRE FOR WELLBEING

6 Hatherley Road
Winchester
Hampshire SO22 6RT
Tel/Fax: 01962 866302
Individual consultations, and courses in connection with the work of Deepak Chopra.

THE YOGA FOR HEALTH FOUNDATION

Ickwell Bury
Biggleswade SG18 9EF
Tel: 01767 627271
Runs training and therapy courses in Yoga and workshops in Ayurveda in beautiful surroundings and a healing environment.

THE AYURVEDIC INSTITUTE

PO Box 23445
Albuquerque, NM 87192-1445
Tel: (505) 291 9698
Fax: (505) 294 7572
Under the directorship of Dr Vasant Lad, the Institute offers the Ayurvedic Studies Program over three trimesters from November to the following June. This is traditional Ayurveda taught in depth. The Institute also runs seminars on related topics like Yoga, Jyotish, Vedic palmistry and Tantra. Also available: private consultations, Pancha Karma treatment, herbs and a correspondence course.

BANYAN TRADING CO.

PO Box 13002
Albuquerque, NM 87192
Tel: (1-800) 953 6424 or (505) 244 1880
Fax: (505) 244 1878
website: www.banyantrading.com
Wholesale only. Traditional Ayurvedic herbs and products.

INTERNATURAL

33719 116th Street
Dept. VL
Twin Lakes, WI 53181
website: www.internatural.com
Supplies Ayurvedic herbs, personal care and healthcare products, tapes and videos, vitamins/supplements and books.

SUSHAKTI

Tel: (970) 259 5587

email: info@ayurveda-sushakti.com

website: www.ayurveda-sushakti.com

Offers Ayurvedic books, herbal and skincare products.

APPENDIX: KICHADI

Kichadi means a bean/grain mixture. Kichadi made of white Basmati rice and split mung beans is particularly easy to digest and very nourishing. This being so it is recommended in Ayurveda when the digestion is poor, or prior to Pancha Karma treatment. Kichadi can be cooked to varying consistencies: the more soup-like, the more easily assimilated.

Vegetables suitable for your Doshic type or to help redress an imbalance can be added to the basic recipe. Root vegetables can be added to the pot with the rice and beans; leafy vegetables can be added towards the end of the cooking period.

RECIPE

SERVES 2–3

INGREDIENTS

½ cup white Basmati rice
¼ cup split yellow mung beans (mung dhal)
1 tablespoon Ghee (clarified butter)
spices (amount to taste, but try as suggested):

1 teaspoon cumin seeds

1 teaspoon coriander seeds

½ teaspoon fennel seeds

1 teaspoon turmeric – these four spices make a blend suitable for all Doshas

¼ teaspoon asafoetida – the addition of this helps Vata digestion and flatulence

1 teaspoon minced root ginger

¼ teaspoon ground black pepper

¼ teaspoon black mustard seeds – adding these three warms the mix considerably for Vata and Kapha Doshas

½ teaspoon salt (sea or rock salt)

6 cups boiling water

vegetables (optional) – asparagus is delicious in Kichadi and is suitable for all three Doshas

the addition of lime and chopped fresh coriander leaves as condiments cools the mix for Pitta Dosha

Wash the rice well to remove excess starch. Wash the split mung beans and pick through them to remove any tiny stones, bits of stalk or discoloured pieces of mung bean.

Melt the ghee in a heavy pan (stainless steel or enamelled cast iron) and add the seeds and heat until they pop, then add the salt, the other spices, rice and split mung beans. Stir well to ensure the newly added ingredients are well-coated in ghee and spices, then add the boiling water to cover the contents of the pan by about 2 inches (5 cm). Simmer until all ingredients are soft, adding more water if necessary. Continue to cook until the desired consistency is reached.

Serve with lime and coriander (as suggested above) for Pitta, with some pickle for Kapha and Vata (who can also have some plain yoghurt with the meal).

Since Ayurveda recommends freshly prepared food to maximize the Prana available, it is best to prepare only enough for one meal at a time.